Low Back Pain

WHAT DO I DO NOW? PAIN MEDICINE

Mark P Jensen and Lynn R. Webster

SERIES EDITORS

Low Back Pain

Edited by

Christopher J. Standaert, MD, MSHCT
Associate Professor, University of Pittsburgh School of Medicine,
Pittsburgh, USA

and

Janna Friedly, MD, MPH
Professor, University of Washington School of Medicine,
Seattle, USA

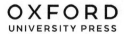

OXFORD
UNIVERSITY PRESS

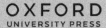

OXFORD
UNIVERSITY PRESS

Oxford University Press is a department of the University of Oxford. It furthers
the University's objective of excellence in research, scholarship, and education
by publishing worldwide. Oxford is a registered trade mark of Oxford University
Press in the UK and certain other countries.

Published in the United States of America by Oxford University Press
198 Madison Avenue, New York, NY 10016, United States of America.

CIP data is on file at the Library of Congress

ISBN 978-0-19-765284-8

DOI: 10.1093/med/9780197652848.001.0001

Printed by Sheridan Books, Inc., United States of America

Contents

Contributors

Derek R. Anderson, PhD, VA Puget Sound – American Lake Division, Tacoma, WA, USA

Steven J. Atlas, MD, MPH, Harvard Medical School, Boston, MA, USA

Robert L. Bailey, MD, University of Pittsburgh, Pittsburgh, PA, USA

Kristina Barber, MD, Colorado Rehabilitation and Occupational Medicine, Greenwood Village, CO, USA

Karen Barr, MD, University of Pittsburgh School of Medicine, Pittsburgh, PA, USA

Seth Bires, DO, Northwestern University/Shirley Ryan Ability Lab, Chicago, IL, USA

Jason S. Bitterman, MD, University of Connecticut, Hartford, CT, USA

Rachel Brakke Holman, MD, University of Colorado School of Medicine, Aurora, CO, USA

Moriah J. Brier, PhD, VISN 20 Clinical Resource Hub, Boise, ID, USA

Kevin A. Carneiro, DO, University Of North Carolina, Chapel Hill, NC, USA

Kuntal Chowdhary, MD, Weill Cornell Medicine, New York, NY, USA

Deborah Crane, MD, MPH, University of Washington, Seattle, WA, USA

Charles B. Davis, MD, Consulting Radiologists, Ltd., Santa Monica, CA, USA

James E. Eubanks, Jr, MD, MS, Medical University of South Carolina, Charleston, SC, USA

Michelle Eventov, MD, Johns Hopkins University, Baltimore, MD, USA

Janna L. Friedly, MD, MPH, University of Washington, Seattle, WA, USA

Christopher Gibbs, MD, University of Pittsburgh Medical Center, Pittsburgh, PA, USA

Ari Greis, DO, Rothman Orthopedic Institute at Thomas Jefferson University, Philadelphia, PA, USA

Mark A. Harrast, MD, University of Washington, Seattle, WA, USA

Erica J. Ho, PhD, VA Puget Sound Health Care System, Seattle, WA, USA

Benjamin D. Holmes, DC, PhD, Mayo Clinic, Rochester, MN, USA

Jeffrey G. Jarvik, MD, MPH, FAAR, University of Washington School of Medicine, Seattle, WA, USA

Prakash Jayabalan, MD, PhD, Northwestern Feinberg School of Medicine, Chicago, IL, USA

Eman Kazi, MD, Warren Alpert Medical School of Brown University, Providence, USA

Mary S. Keszler, MD, Johns Hopkins University School of Medicine, Baltimore, MD, USA

Rupali Kumar, MD, University of Texas Southwestern Medical Center, Dallas, Texas, USA

Laura R. Lawson, MD, Richmond VA Medical Center, Richmond, VA, USA

Isaiah Levy, MD, University of Pittsburgh, Pittsburgh, PA, USA

Marissa L. Marcotte, MD, University of Washington, Seattle, WA, USA

Niveditha Mohan, MD, University of Pittsburgh, Pittsburgh, PA, USA

David C. Morgenroth, MD, University of Washington, Seattle, WA, USA

Anthony A. Oyekan, MD, University of Pittsburgh Medical Center, Pittsburgh, PA, USA

Charles A. Reitman, MD, Medical University of South Carolina, Charleston, SC, USA

Dominic Ridolfi, MD, Northwestern University, Chicago, IL, USA

Eric J. Roseen, DC, MSc, Boston University Chobanian & Avedisian School of Medicine, Boston, MA, USA

Michael J. Schneider, DC, PhD, University of Pittsburgh, Pittsburgh, PA, USA

Jeremy D. Shaw, MD, Intermountain Health, Salt Lake City, USA

Joseph P. Shivers, MD, University of Pittsburgh School of Medicine, Pittsburgh, PA, USA

Katharine Smolinski, DO, University of Utah, Salt Lake City, USA

Christopher J. Standaert, MD, MSHCT, University of Pittsburgh School of Medicine, Pittsburgh, PA, USA

Jaxon E. Standaert, Ohio State University, Columbus, OH, USA

Jessica Sullivan, PA-C, MPAS, University of Pittsburgh Medical Center, Pittsburgh, PA, USA

William Taylor Riden, DO, MBA, University of Tennessee, Knoxville, TN, USA

Laura M. Tuck, PsyD, VA Puget Sound Healthcare System, Seattle, WA, USA

Aaron P. Turner, PhD, VA Puget Sound Health Care System, Seattle, WA, USA

Maria A. Vanushkina, MD, UCHealth, Colorado Springs, CO, USA

Alex Watson, MD, MBA, Admire Medical, Middletown, DE, USA

Debra K. Weiner, MD, University of Pittsburgh, Pittsburgh, PA, USA

Rhonda M. Williams, PhD, VA Puget Sound Health Care System, Seattle, WA, USA

Introduction: We Need to Think Differently About Low Back Pain

The care of low back pain (LBP) is plagued by variability, a lack of guideline-based care, over-medicalization of biopsychosocial problems, inequity, and an overemphasis on interventional and operative care. There are also significant problems related to our understanding of and our published literature on LBP. Guidelines focused on the short-term management of acute LBP are generally not followed by clinicians and have limited applicability in clinical care. The reality is that LBP, as a singular entity, is a chronic recurrent problem for most individuals. Care should therefore be directed toward a chronic disease management model, focusing on optimizing function and long-term health.

Importantly for this book, all LBP conditions are also not created equally. "Low back pain" is a symptom, not a diagnosis, and is analogous to symptoms like shortness of breath and abdominal pain. There are a number of specific conditions that can be related to or causal of LBP, and there are a host of comorbidities that influence natural history and care. Disc herniations, degenerative spinal stenosis, and tumors may all cause radicular pain and radiculopathy, but natural history and treatment considerations are clearly different. Isthmic spondylolisthesis is not the same as degenerative spondylolisthesis, either in demographics, natural history, or treatment considerations. Chronic LBP in patients with anxiety and depression requires a different approach to similar symptoms in those without associated mental health issues, as treatment of comorbid conditions and response to specific treatment approaches are different. Failure to recognize specific conditions, such as a far lateral disc herniation in an older adult, ankylosing spondylitis in a young adult, or hip pathology, can lead to inappropriate treatment and unnecessary suffering for patients. The approach to LBP in those with widespread pain, medical frailty, pregnancy, work-related injuries, and obesity is also different from those with isolated low back issues. Nonspecific and poorly verified diagnoses further confound treatment approaches. Marginalization, psychological trauma, bias, and ethnocultural and socioeconomic factors affect care at all levels. Many aspects of spine care are also controversial, including the treatment of fractures, spinal stenosis, and disc herniations.

How do medical providers, much less the patients and general public, make sense of all of this? By using actual clinical presentations, this book helps to accomplish this. There are chapters focusing on acute and chronic

LBP, but others go deeper in considering the effects of specific sports, like golf and running, or specific comorbid conditions like depression, obesity, spinal cord injury, amputation, pregnancy, and frailty. Examples of the critical "red flag" conditions of traumatic fracture, tumor, infection, and cauda equina syndrome are included, as are cases covering pathologies like compression fracture and spondylolysis. Common structural issues, like disc herniations, spinal stenosis, spondylolisthesis, and scoliosis, are also discussed. All cases present the essential steps of diagnosis and initial management, generally delving deeper to outline more advanced care, differential outcomes, and equity. All take a critical approach to the existing data to dispel common misconceptions, identify ineffective care, and provide the best possible advice on diagnosis and treatment.

The information presented here will help primary care and other providers develop a structured approach to care and effectively manage a range of common clinical situations. The depth included will be of use to physical medicine and rehabilitation (PM&R) specialists, surgeons, physical therapists, chiropractic providers, rheumatologists, and others in addressing a wide range of conditions. The authors provide expertise across the spectrum of care and include specialists in PM&R, orthopedic and neurological surgery, chiropractic, rheumatology, geriatrics, sports medicine, radiology, and psychology, along with established researchers in an array of related fields.

The cases in this book provide clarity on numerous conditions, delineate known natural histories and clinical features, and take a critical approach to the application of all forms of care. Over the entire population of those with LBP and related disorders, the role for surgery and interventional spine care is limited. The overwhelming majority of patients can and should be managed with education, activity modifications, psychologically informed care, appropriate but not excessive diagnostic evaluation, and appropriate support. With a better understanding of some of the various conditions that exist under the broader rubric of "low back pain," primary care providers and others should be more comfortable and capable of assisting their patients and directing them toward appropriate care.

1 "Should I Go to the Emergency Room?": Their First Episode of Low Back Pain

Christopher J. Standaert

A 32-year-old calls your office with a concern of acute low back pain (LBP). The symptoms started this morning. The patient states they just bent forward to brush their teeth, and their "back went out." They report severe axial LBP across the lower lumbar area with no radiation into either leg. It is difficult to stand up straight, and the pain is a bit better laying supine on the floor. This has never happened before. There is no weakness, numbness, bladder change, or other neurologic symptoms. The patient has no history of other significant medical problems, has had no surgery, and takes no prescription medications. There was no trauma, and the patient has had no fever, recent illness, or other similar concerns. The patient is a customer service representative at a nearby company and did not go to work today.

They ask if they should come to your office or go to an emergency room. They also ask for a medication prescription or other suggestions to help with the pain.

What do you do now?

Acute LBP is a common clinical symptom affecting almost every person at some point in their life. Lifetime prevalence is reported to be 85%, likely an underestimation, and about 7% of patients in a primary care practice see their medical provider for LBP in any given year. Although the majority of acute episodes of LBP are self-limiting, recurrent pain occurs in about 50–75% of individuals within 1 year, and only a minority of patients are actually fully recovered and pain free at 1 year. Further complicating this, about half of patients presenting to a clinician for acute LBP actually have a history of prior LBP. Clinical guidelines tend to incorrectly address acute LBP as a self-limiting condition. For the majority of patients, LBP is a chronic-recurrent disease, and patients need to be approached with this in mind, meaning that clinicians need to consider the potential long-term consequences for their patients. This influences initial treatment recommendations but also the use of language, addressing expectations and fear, the need to focus on long-term active approaches to health and well-being, and recognizing that many have prior experiences with LBP—often negative ones.

The primary goals of treatment for acute LBP center on maintaining mobility and restoring prior level of function. Acute interventions for pain that either are associated with adverse long-term consequences, such as opioid medications, or that foster passivity on the part of the patient, such as excessive rest and withdrawal from work and social contacts, can be detrimental and are best avoided. Active therapy, such as exercise, stretching, and adaptive work or home strategies, tend to offer more benefit. Exercise is the only treatment that has been shown to reduce the rate of future occurrences of LBP.

Taking an appropriate history in those with acute LBP includes a screen for "red flag" conditions, a discussion about the nature of the symptoms and any injury and prior experiences with LBP, a review of the general medical history, and a review of beliefs, work-related issues, and psychosocial factors that may elevate the risk of transition to chronic pain ("yellow flags"). "Red flag" conditions include fracture, tumor, infection, and severe neurological injury. Screening for these is challenging, as about 80% of patients will have a symptom or historical feature correlating with a red flag condition. Clearly, all of these patients will not warrant urgent medical evaluation. Red flag symptoms by themselves are not an indication for spinal imaging;

nor is their absence a contraindication to imaging. These decisions have to be made in the entire context of the patient's situation. That said, some symptoms or historical features are more helpful than others. A prior history of cancer is the best predictive factor for cancer. Fever, immunosuppression, intravenous drug use, and the use of corticosteroids are the best predictors of infection; and major trauma in a younger individual or minor trauma in someone with a high risk for or known osteoporosis is the most important indicator of possible fracture.

Given that about half of patients presenting with acute LBP have had LBP before, it is important to review any prior experience with LBP that the patient may have had. They should be asked about how they approached prior episodes, what helped or did not help, if they returned to baseline function and activities, and if they are afraid of anything in particular. It is problematic if they express poor outcomes from prior episodes, loss of function, fear, and the use of passive approaches like medications, ultrasound therapy, and rest. These previous experiences may suggest that their expectation for recovery in this episode is similar and predict a poor outcome, high risk of further injury, and a desire for passive care.

It is critical to address fear as this is what often drives the disability associated with LBP. Patients may well fear that they have sustained significant harm, have a severe underlying condition, or that their spine is fragile and at risk of further injury with activity. Beliefs of this type need to be addressed at the initial visit with reassurance and encouragement to stay active and work through any functional restrictions or fears, with the guidance of physical therapy or other providers as indicated.

An exploration of "yellow flags" should be part of the routine evaluation of those with LBP. These are psychosocial factors that are associated with a poor outcome from acute pain and a subsequent transition to chronic pain. Depression, anxiety, social withdrawal, a history of physical, sexual, or psychological abuse, and a history of perceived injustice and marginalization are affective factors associated with poor outcomes from acute LBP. Several work-related issues similarly predict poor outcomes, including job dissatisfaction, perception of a poor or hostile work environment, a short duration of employment in a current position, and an absence of light duty work for those sustaining injury. Importantly, being a member of an ethnocultural minority or marginalized group is also associated with poor outcomes, potentially related to differential access to care, provider bias, distrust in the health care system, language barriers, financial barriers, or other socioeconomic factors. Belief systems, such as fear avoidance (avoiding specific activities due to a fear of further harm), catastrophizing (an amplified version of fear avoidance with exaggerated fear about the worst possible outcomes from activity or future events), and a passive coping style are all clearly associated with worse outcomes for those with acute LBP.

Physical examination in those with acute LBP is similarly intended to address red flag conditions and to get some sense of the patient's limitations and needs. The presence of a fever is concerning for infection. Gait should be observed, including heel and toe walking. It is important to look at and palpate the lumbar spine. Focal tenderness and/or bruising in those at risk of fracture is concerning. Flank pain and tenderness may be suggestive of a renal issue. Lumbar spine range of motion is done within what is comfortable for the patient. Data on normal range of motion are lacking, so the intention is to see what the patient is able or willing to do. Hip range of motion should also be assessed, given the overlap of hip and lumbar spine symptoms. Neurologic exam focuses on lower extremity strength, sensation, and reflexes at the patellae and ankles. Clear neurologic loss is concerning and should prompt more rapid evaluation. Consistency between the history and the exam findings is important. Inconsistencies are often seen in those with a psychosocial component to their situation.

Diagnostic imaging is not indicated for acute LBP absent red flag concerns. Excessive imaging tends to complicate care unnecessarily and is associated with worse outcomes. As people age, the prevalence of "abnormalities" on imaging become very common in the normal population, including disc height loss, spondylolisthesis, disc bulging, spinal stenosis, and even disc herniations. The significance of any of these in the setting of acute LBP is questionable, and they are likely unrelated to the presenting symptoms. Laboratory studies can be obtained if there are red flag concerns or if there is concern for an underlying medical disorder that is not strictly related to the lumbar spine. This is not indicated for uncomplicated LBP with no indication of a concerning process.

Effective treatment centers on advice to maintain activity within tolerance and to pursue light, low-impact aerobic activity like walking or swimming, limiting bed rest and the use of oral medications and imaging, and avoiding the iatrogenic disability associated with the use of opiates, excessive functional limitations, and negative language (including "degenerative disc disease," "you have a bad back," and "don't do anything that hurts"). Clinicians also need to avoid creating false diagnostic narratives as to what the problem may be. We simply do not know the cause of acute LBP in almost all patients, and telling patients that it is a "sprain," "pulled muscle," "slipped disc" or similar may result in unwarranted beliefs about the severity of injury and future implications. Phrases like "I have no reason to think anything bad has happened to your back," "there is no indication of a significant structural injury," or "this can get better if you keep moving and work through it" may be more effective. The prime objective is to foster a return to function and healthy behaviors and not to limit future function or generate fear or beliefs of frailty.

Despite widespread use, there is little evidence to support the use of medications in acute LBP. There is some evidence supporting a mild benefit from nonsteroidal anti-inflammatory drugs (NSAIDs) and skeletal muscle relaxants, although there are also well-documented side effects associated with these. There are clear data that acetaminophen and anticonvulsants (such as gabapentinoids) are *ineffective*, and these should generally not be used, particularly given the potential side effects for anticonvulsants. There is no evidence to support the use of corticosteroids for acute LBP. Any short-term relief associated with the use of opiates is of doubtful clinical significance, and there are no data supporting long-term use or benefit. Given the high rate of adverse effects and opioid dependence or addiction, these drugs should generally be avoided in acute LBP. The Centers for Disease Control has found that a single 10-day prescription of opiates is associated with a 20% probability that the person receiving that prescription will still be taking opiates 1 year later. Multiple studies of patients seen for acute LBP in emergency departments have found no added benefit to giving patients opioids, benzodiazepines, or muscle relaxants in addition to NSAIDs.

Spinal manipulation is commonly pursued by those with acute LBP. However, the evidence of benefit is lacking. There are some data suggesting a very small benefit from manipulation but no evidence of any long-term benefit. There is also no evidence that manipulation is superior to any other treatment, such as exercise. Topical heat can be helpful in the setting of acute LBP. Excessive rest is clearly harmful.

Exercise is generally the best supported treatment for LBP, although there are no real data to suggest that any one particular approach is uniquely beneficial. It is clear that those who remain physically active in the setting of acute LBP have better outcomes than those who do not. There is also evidence that addressing fear-avoidant beliefs early in the treatment course is important in optimizing outcomes, and this can be incorporated into advice to remain active or structured training through physical therapy. Referrals for physical therapy for acute LBP should recommend therapeutic exercise and the avoidance of passive care, like ultrasound. Ultimately, the most effective exercise is one that the patient will do. This could be cardiovascular exercise like walking or swimming, modified yoga, or exercises prescribed by physical therapists. There is no specific exercise that anyone has to do to improve, so it is best to take a very flexible approach to exercise and activity. Being excessively dogmatic about any specific approach is not consistent with the evidence and is likely harmful in those with a higher risk of chronicity, as they are less likely to follow through with recommended exercise. These patients need to be successful in an initial exercise program, requiring an individualized approach.

There is very little if any information available on differential treatment courses based on gender or ethnocultural identity. However, it is clear that women, Blacks, and those of low socioeconomic status with pain are fundamentally treated differently than males, Caucasians, or wealthier individuals, respectively. Clinical practice guidelines generally fail to differentiate recommendations along any of these lines. Lived experience with pain, injustice, trauma, or marginalization may influence how a given individual responds to pain and interacts with the health care system. Providers need to be aware of these issues and of their own unconscious biases so that they can help their patient achieve the best outcome.

Given this, how do we address the patient presented in the case above? This patient has no red flag concerns in their history. If they are able to stand, walk, and perform basic activities of daily living, they do not necessarily need a formal medical evaluation. They can be assured that these symptoms are likely to diminish or resolve within a week or so and that the best way to achieve that is to stay active, performing short bouts of movement or activity routinely throughout the day or engaging in routine, low-impact aerobic exercise if that is what they were doing before the onset of their LBP. They should also be advised to resume regular activities as they improve. Given their age and general health, it is reasonable to recommend the use of over-the-counter NSAIDs. If these cannot be tolerated, or the patient cannot sleep due to pain, a skeletal muscle relaxant could be prescribed. Topical heat can be recommended. Given the absence of red flag concerns, there is no indication to go to the emergency department for evaluation unless the patient is unable to care for themselves. There is also no need for X-rays or other spinal imaging. If the patient's symptoms do not resolve over a week or so, or if they want to learn some stretching or exercise approaches for their back, physical therapy can be prescribed. If the patient can work through this situation and resume their activities, there is no need for physical therapy. Any language expressed reflecting fear avoidance should be met with reassurance and advice to move. This event may well occur again, so equipping the patient with confidence in their capacity for self-care is important. Helping this patient with developing a regular exercise program is the best way to minimize recurrences. A summary of the "dos and don'ts" of managing acute LBP is in Box 1.1.

BOX 1.1 **Do's and Don'ts for Acute Low Back Pain**

Do

Screen for red flags:

Fracture

Tumor

Infection

Significant neurologic loss

Screen for yellow flags/psychosocial risk factors:

Fear

Anxiety/depression

History of abuse/trauma

Social/cultural marginalization

Adverse work/employment factors

Job dissatisfaction

Lack of light duty work

Limited duration of employment

Perform a physical examination:

Gait/observation

Palpation/range of motion (within tolerance)

Neurological examination

Hip examination

Encourage activity/movement

Use positive language:

"This is likely to get better soon, especially if you keep moving."

"I am not worried that anything bad has happened to your back."

Consider topical heat, NSAIDs, and muscle relaxants

Consider physical therapy for guided exercise or if not improving

Encourage light duty work if job function is affected

Don't

Tell patients to rest excessively or discourage mild activity

Order imaging without clear indications of significant pathology

Ignore their emotional/psychosocial state or fear

Use negative language or provide presumptive structural explanations:

"You have a bad back."

"It is probably a slipped disc."

"Don't do anything that hurts."

Routinely prescribe acetaminophen, anticonvulsants/gabapentinoids, opiates, or benzodiazepines

Emphasize the use of passive approaches like rest, electrical stimulation, or braces

Remove or restrict from all work if light duty options exist

1. Although most episodes of acute LBP are self-limiting, recurrence rates are extremely high, and most people do not fully recover at 1 year. LBP is thus best approached as a chronic, recurrent disorder.
2. Psychosocial and affective factors are the best predictors of an episode of acute LBP transitioning to a chronic pain state. These include depression, anxiety, trauma, social marginalization, passive coping, and fear.
3. The primary goal of treatment for acute LBP is to help a patient return to their baseline level of function.
4. Exercise is the best supported treatment for acute LBP, and patients should be encouraged to remain active and engage in progressive exercise.
5. Excessive rest, unnecessary imaging, negative language, inaccurate and unhelpful diagnoses, excessive activity restrictions, and reliance on generally unhelpful or overtly harmful medications lead to iatrogenic disability and worse outcomes.

Further reading

1. Kreiner DS, Matz P, Bono CM, et al. Guideline summary review: an evidence-based clinical guideline for the diagnosis and treatment of low back pain. Spine J. 2020 Jul;20(7):998–1024. doi: 10.1016/j.spinee.2020.04.006. Epub 2020 Apr 22. Erratum in: Spine J. 2021 Feb 24; PMID: 32333996.
2. Skolasky RL, Maggard AM, Thorpe RJ Jr, Wegener ST, Riley LH 3rd. United States hospital admissions for lumbar spinal stenosis: racial and ethnic differences, 2000 through 2009. Spine (Phila Pa 1976). 2013 Dec 15;38(26):2272–2278. doi: 10.1097/BRS.0b013e3182a3d392. PMID: 23873234.
3. Strudwick K, McPhee M, Bell A, Martin-Khan M, Russell T. Review article: best practice management of low back pain in the emergency department (part 1 of the musculoskeletal injuries rapid review series). Emerg Med Australas. 2018 Feb;30(1):18–35. doi: 10.1111/1742-6723.12907. Epub 2017 Dec 12. PMID: 29232762.
4. Verhagen AP, Downie A, Popal N, Maher C, Koes BW. Red flags presented in current low back pain guidelines: a review. Eur Spine J. 2016 Sep;25(9):2788–2802. doi: 10.1007/s00586-016-4684-0. Epub 2016 Jul 4. PMID: 27376890.

2 "My Back Went Out Again!": You Are Seeing Them at 1:00

Karen Barr

Your 1:00 patient has already been in to see you three times this year for "flares" of low back pain and is coming in again today with the same concerns. Each prior episode this year has resolved over a couple of weeks, only to recur a few months later. Your patient has become steadily more distressed about the back pain each time. When starting the visit at 1:00, your patient reports another "flare" of non-radiating low back pain. They seem anxious and concerned about the recurrent events. Each episode has started with normal everyday activities. The patient does not exercise and, at this point, is rather sedentary and avoids routine household and yard tasks. The patient is 41 years old and otherwise healthy except for stable hypertension. The pain is interrupting their work in sales, as it has been hard to sit or stand long for a few days with each event. They ask if you can give them anything to make the pain stay away or if they need surgery.

What do you do now?

Although recurrence of low back pain can be distressing to patients, it is actually the norm medically. Systematic reviews estimate that somewhere between a third and three-fourths of people who experience acute low back pain (LBP) will have at least one recurrence of LBP in the following year, and most continue to have episodes of significant pain and disability in the future. A systematic approach to the evaluation of episodic back pain, management of comorbidities associated with back pain, and patient education (to mitigate risk factors for recurrence and teach self-management strategies) can reduce the health care costs associated with this very common symptom and decrease disability in patients.

A thoughtful evaluation can reduce the risk of over-medicalization and excessive disability. In patients with LBP, it is rare for the specific cause to be identified, and the fact that it is recurrent does not make identification more likely or make it necessary to pursue a specific cause. Of course, having benign LBP in the past is not protective of acquiring a serious cause of LBP in the future, so it is wise to adhere to a strategy that uses a combination of patient history and physical exam to identify potential causes that might require specific treatment. In this case, there are no features of the case that make a serious cause of back pain likely. The patient has no neurological symptoms in the legs. They have not experienced a trauma that could have caused a fracture, do not have known risk factors for osteoporosis, and do not have a history of malignancy, autoimmune disease, or increased risk for infection, such as intravenous drug use or recent medical procedure to the spine. They have no worrisome symptoms such as unexplained weight loss, fevers, or symptoms concerning for rheumatological disease. A normal physical exam would give added reassurance.

This methodical approach can assure both the practitioner and the patient that nothing serious has been missed. It also helps to avoid the overuse of imaging and medical interventions. The risk for over-medicalization in cases such as this is real. The United States has the highest direct medical costs in the world for the treatment of LBP but does not have better outcomes than other countries. This is known as the "low back pain paradox": unnecessary medical investigations can lead to expensive but ineffective and potentially harmful health care and paradoxically increase the risk of long-term, back-related disability. The pressure to "do something" can feel intense, but it can lead to real harm, so it should be resisted. For example, ordering imaging that is not indicated often leads to diagnostic jargon on imaging reports that feeds a patient's fear and belief that their spine is seriously damaged but cannot be fixed. This can be further compounded by language that physicians use to explain these findings, such as "degeneration" which have been shown to worsen fear avoidance and therefore can increase disability.

This approach of careful assessment followed by patient education can also begin to educate the patient on ways they can assess and manage their own back pain by distinguishing between features of back pain that would necessitate further investigation and features that are benign in nature and can be managed without medical intervention. The practitioner's attention to the patient's concerns, and reassurance that nothing serious has been missed, can help reduce the patient's anxiety.

In this case, the patient asks if there is "anything to make the pain stay away." Risk factors for recurrent or persistent LBP have been identified, and patient education to reduce modifiable risk factors may motivate them to adopt a healthier lifestyle. Unhealthy health habits as a whole appear to cluster together as a risk factor for the development for LBP, even when controlled for age and body mass index (BMI).

Proven healthy behaviors that patients can adopt to decrease risk of recurrence or chronicity of LBP include not smoking, being at a healthy weight, and engaging in physical exercise. Smoking increases the risk of both recurrent LBP and of LBP becoming chronic. Excess weight is another modifiable risk factor. The risk of LBP increases as BMI rises. The risk of chronic LBP is about 3% in patients with normal BMI, 5% in overweight people, nearly 8% in obese patients, and nearly 12% in very obese patients (see chapter 33 for a discussion of LBP and obesity). Physical activity seems to mitigate the effects of weight, with the biggest benefits of exercise on the incidence of LBP occurring in overweight and obese patients. Multiple studies have demonstrated that exercise reduces the risk of recurrent episodes of LBP. A sedentary lifestyle and increased sitting time have also been associated with increases in recurrent and chronic LBP. Reassurance that routine household and yard tasks (other than very heavy lifting) do not contribute to recurrent LBP, but are, in fact, very likely to contribute to a better outcome, can be comforting.

Low social support, social isolation, worry, and stress are associated with persistent pain and should be frankly discussed so they can be addressed if possible. A major comorbidity associated with persistent LBP and pain-related disability is depression, seen in 30–50% of patients with persistent pain. Multiple studies have found depression to be significantly associated with poor outcomes. Depression makes it particularly difficult to self-manage pain, so detecting the presence of depression and appropriately treating it can be a crucial step in managing recurrent episodes of back pain.

Patients should be specifically counseled that there is no surgery, injection, or medication that can prevent future episodes of pain—the best tools we have to prevent future episodes are exercise, avoiding being too sedentary, and healthy lifestyle choices, such as not smoking and achieving a healthy BMI.

A person's behavior and beliefs can have a significant impact on back pain chronicity. LBP-induced functional limitations can become coupled with beliefs. Patients become fearful that activity will cause pain, leading to a downward spiral of limiting activity because of fear of pain, and gradually become disabled because of deconditioning and fear. Fear avoidance beliefs have been linked to subacute back pain becoming chronic as well as linked to more pain and disability during acute episodes of back pain. Even the patient's belief that they are at high risk for persistent pain is a risk factor for this to become true. A number of psychosocial factors associated with persistent pain, often termed "yellow flags," are delineated in Table 2.1.

Information in the case that the patient is becoming steadily more distressed with each episode of back pain and their reduction in activity raises concern that they could be falling into this fear avoidance spiral. There is good evidence that patients with fear avoidance beliefs do better if these beliefs are addressed rather than ignored. Treatments shown to be effective include advice to be active and discussion of fear avoidance and psychological concerns and would be a good start for this patient. Other effective strategies are graded activity increases (increasing activity in a planned, graded fashion without over-attention to symptoms), psychologically informed physical therapy, and (if these thoughts are becoming pervasive) cognitive behavioral therapy.

TABLE 2.1 Yellow Flags. Psychosocial Factors Associated with Chronic Pain

Belief structures

Fear avoidance

Catastrophizing

Passive coping style

High level of illness conviction

Self-perceived poor health

Low expectation of improvement

Withdrawal from social interactions

Poor adherence to exercise or self-care

Mood/affective factors

Depression

Anxiety

Irritability

Sleep disturbance

History of trauma or abuse

Somatization

Substance use disorder

Occupational factors

Prolonged time off from work

Absence of light duty work

Low level of education

Short duration of employment in current position

Poor job satisfaction

Perception of poor work environment

There is strong evidence that self-management programs are effective in improving symptoms of LBP, improving functional status, and reducing psychological distress. These differ from passive patient education material because they emphasize patient skill development to manage symptoms, make lifestyle changes, and promote self-efficacy. Typical problem-solving around self-management include learning skills to cope with fear and other negative emotions, goal setting, stress management techniques (such as mindfulness and deep breathing), strategies to increase physical activity, sleep hygiene, and coaching in how to communicate preferences to providers. Facilitators of pain self-management found in qualitative studies include treatment of depression if present, support of family, friends, medical staff, and peers, goal setting, adoption of positive thinking, and being provided with a menu of different strategies to use.

In this case, teaching self-management begins with a discussion to uncover the patient's beliefs about their back (such as if they believe it is damaged), so that they can be addressed, and an open discussion of fear, distress, and ways to cope with these negative emotions and stress. Coaching the patient to set goals regarding activity and fitness, which includes regular exercise, and clear communication that movement is better than rest for their back (both to prevent recurrence and during a flare), can counteract fear avoidant beliefs. If the patient is not confident that they can begin and maintain an exercise program or make other necessary lifestyle changes, resources to help them should be explored.

A menu of options to decrease symptoms if pain does recur should include non-pharmacological/nonmedical treatment options like heat, massage, gentle stretches, foam roller, a standing desk at work to allow for easy changes in position, and similar strategies. Having these options available could increase the patient's confidence that they have the tools necessary to deal with their back pain when it recurs.

KEY POINTS

1. The natural history of LBP is one of recurrent episodes, and therefore a recurrence alone is not a reason to suspect serious pathology.

2. Many of the risk factors for transition to chronic LBP can be reduced with lifestyle modifications and attention to mental health.
3. Distress and fear of pain in themselves are contributors to LBP and disability, and addressing these aspects is part of an effective management strategy.
4. Teaching techniques to self-manage recurrent LBP and facilitating the use of these strategies is an effective way to reduce overutilization of health care and decrease back-related disability and pain.
5. Exercise, goals for activity, belief in success, and good health-directed behavior are essential self-management tools for recurrent LBP.

Further reading

1. Foster NE, Anema JR, Cherkin D, et al. Prevention and treatment of low back pain: evidence, challenges, and promising directions. Lancet. 2018;391(10137):2368–2383.
2. Nicholas MK, Linton SJ, Watson PJ, Main CJ. Early identification and management of psychological risk factors ("yellow flags") in patients with low back pain: a reappraisal. Phys Ther. 2011;91(5):737–753.
3. Wertli MM, Rasmussen-Barr E, Weiser S, Bachmann LM, Brunner F, et al. The role of fear avoidance beliefs as a prognostic factor for outcome in patients with nonspecific low back pain: a systematic review. Spine J. 2014;14(5):816–836.e4.
4. Huang R, Ning J, Chuter VH, et al. Exercise alone and exercise combined with education both prevent episodes of low back pain and related absenteeism: systematic review and network meta-analysis of randomised controlled trials (RCTs) aimed at preventing back pain. Br J Sports Med. 2020;54(13):766–770.
5. Steffens D, Maher CG, Pereira LSM, et al. Prevention of Low Back Pain: A Systematic Review and Meta-analysis. JAMA Intern Med. 2016;176(2):199–208.
6. Bair MJ, Matthias MS, Nyland RA, et al. Barriers and facilitators to chronic pain self-management: a qualitative study of primary care patients with comorbid musculoskeletal pain and depression. Pain Med. 2009;10(7):1280–1290.

3 "It Hurts Right There.": Focal, Ongoing Back Pain in a 48-Year-Old

Christopher J. Standaert

A 48-year-old female comes in for evaluation for her back pain. This has been occurring daily for 3 years and seems to be activity-related. It is highly focal, and she points to her left lower lumbar area as the location of her pain. There is no pain or paresthesia into her legs. The pain bothers her at work. She has worked as a server at a local restaurant for 15 years. She is a single mother of three children and feels like her job and home demands provide a significant amount of physical activity. She does not exercise beyond this. She went to physical therapy a few years ago but did not do the exercises and does not remember them. She takes 400 mg of ibuprofen 3 or 4 times per day for her pain. A report of X-rays from 1 year ago notes loss of disc height at L4/5 and facet arthropathy in the lower lumbar spine. She thinks there must be something wrong with her lower left spine and asks if it can be "fixed."

What do you do now?

In general, it is very difficult to definitively diagnose a singular cause of low back pain (LBP) in the majority of people presenting for clinical care. Theoretically, any structure in the spine that has a nerve supply can cause pain, including the vertebrae, intervertebral discs, associated joints ("facet" or "zygapophyseal" joints), ligaments, muscles, and tendons, along with the nerves themselves. To complicate matters, all of the structures at a given anatomic level are derived from the same embryologic origin and share similar patterns of pain representation in the central nervous system. This means that pain arising from a vertebra or ligament or joint at a given level occurs in a similar location. It is thus very hard, if not impossible, for patients or clinicians to determine what structure is causing pain simply based upon location. This can be very difficult for patients to accept at times, as the location of the pain may seem quite obvious to them.

In patients with significant psychosocial stressors, there may also be some "amplification" or fear associated with the pain that reinforces the perceived importance of identifying a singular structural cause, which is also tied to the expectation or hope that there is a "cure" or "fix" for the problem. Clinicians have to understand and communicate the limitations in our diagnostic ability and in our ability to really "fix" the cause of spinal pain. Although some injuries clearly improve dramatically with time, such as a muscular strain, disc herniation, or fracture, there is no good evidence that medical interventions reliably "fix" the spine and completely absolve patients of their pain. For the majority of patients, helping them effectively manage their activities, health, expectations, and fear around their spine becomes the central goal.

There are numerous studies on pain referral patterns from various structures in the lumbar spine. These are largely performed by provoking a given structure with a mechanical or chemical irritant, like a needle, and mapping out the location of pain perceived by a series of subjects. Intervertebral discs and various joints are most amenable to this type of procedure. As might be predicted by embryology, there is significant overlap between the patterns of pain provocation from structures at the same anatomic level. For example, the L5/S1 disc and facet joint both commonly refer pain to the ipsilateral buttock, which is often confused with pain from the sacrum or pelvic musculature.

Additional components of the history can help clinicians with diagnosis to a degree but are not typically reliable either. Pain from an intervertebral disc is generally considered to be worse with sitting than standing and increased by coughing, sneezing, or other Valsalva maneuvers. However, these are not particularly reliable diagnostic tools, and there are no clear diagnostic criteria for or validated means of diagnosing "discogenic" pain. Similarly, the facet joints (the articulation of the inferior articular process of one vertebra with the superior articular process of the vertebra below it) have been widely studied as a potential source of pain. Pain from these joints is often considered to increase with standing or extending and rotating the lumbar spine. Unfortunately, this is not a valid assumption either, and there are currently no reliable means of diagnosing LBP from a facet joint by any combination of patient history or physical examination. The same holds true for the sacroiliac joint. There are no physical examination, historical, or radiographic features that can accurately diagnose pain arising from the sacroiliac joint (aside from, perhaps, in true inflammatory sacroiliitis; see chapter 30).

When one also considers that we have no reliable means of permanently resolving pain from any spinal structures, it is generally more harmful than helpful to tell patients that they have discogenic, facet, or sacroiliac pain as we do not know that such a statement is true or that we can "fix" the problem. Creating a convenient but false biological or structural narrative with an associated expectation of a cure is detrimental for the physical and emotional well-being of patients. It also can lead to an extensive, wasteful, and potentially harmful search for that cure.

Imaging poses similar problems for clinicians and patients. The patient in the case above is 48 years old and has X-rays showing a loss of disc height with degenerative changes in her facet joints. Given the persistence and focality of her pain, there is a natural assumption that these findings are related to her pain. Perhaps she has "degenerative disc disease" or painful facet joints. The term "degenerative disc disease" is simply not accurate and should disappear from our lexicon. What we see as the manifestations of disc degeneration on imaging are simply the natural effects of aging, hence there is no "disease." In studies on a cohort of patients from the Framingham Heart Study, almost 2/3 of the participants (with a mean age of 52) had disc degeneration and facet arthropathy on computed tomography

(CT). The highest prevalence of facet arthritic changes was seen at L4/5, and there was no association between the presence of degenerative changes in the disc level or facet joints and the presence of LBP. On a population basis, images of the spine in 48-year-olds simply do not look like images in 18-year-olds. This is an easy concept for patients to comprehend.

History, physical examination, and spinal imaging are helpful in sorting out significant pathology (such as a fracture or infection), identifying the presence or absence of involvement of neurological structures, and identifying some specific pathology that may influence care (such as a scoliosis, spondyloarthropathy, an arthritic hip, or a spondylolisthesis). However, these same approaches are unfortunately not particularly helpful in identifying a source of pain. Clinicians then have to consider the risk/cost vs. the benefit in pursuing the "source" of pain or what is often called a "pain generator." Do we subject our patient to a variety of interventional procedures or expansive imaging to accomplish this? For the most part, the term "pain generator" is unhelpful, as it implies that we can find a singular source of pain and then attribute a patient's pain, suffering, and loss of function to that structure. If we then "fix" it, the patient should be better. For the overwhelming majority of patients, this is also a false narrative. Like "degenerative disc disease," the term "pain generator" should disappear from our lexicon.

Despite this, for patients with no medically or neurologically concerning features and imaging showing nonspecific, age-related changes, interventional options will often be considered to identify and treat the source of pain. These include procedures like epidural steroid injections, facet joint injections, and radiofrequency ablation (RFA) of sensory nerves arising from a facet joint. There is no data to support the use of epidural steroid injections for axial LBP (as opposed to radicular pain), and they should not be performed in a patient such as the one in this case with isolated LBP. Injections of corticosteroids into the lumbar facet joints are poorly studied and not supported by the literature. They also should not be routinely used in the treatment of axial LBP.

RFA for facet joints is being utilized with increasing frequency in the treatment of LBP. This procedure involves applying heat generated in a needle tip through the use of radiofrequency current to essentially cauterize or ablate the nerves that carry sensation arising from the facet joint. By ablating the nerves, the joint can theoretically be made insensate for a time until the nerve regenerates, often in 6 to 12 months. Prior to this procedure, patients will generally undergo a series of "diagnostic blocks" in which a small amount of anesthetic is placed in the region of the medial branch nerves associated with a given facet to see if the patient's pain is alleviated. Given very high false positive rates for this procedure (meaning that the block and pain resolution are unrelated), many practitioners perform (and guidelines suggest) multiple confirmatory blocks. As with many medical procedures, the enthusiasm for performing RFA has vastly outstripped the development of evidence supporting its use. There is no high-level evidence that RFA improves pain or function in those with LBP. Even the limited supporting literature shows benefit in only a very small fraction of those potentially eligible for the procedure. Given the high prevalence of LBP and poor evidence of benefit, RFA should also not be routinely pursued in those with persistent axial LBP.

Getting back to the patient presented above, she is 48 years old, has a physically demanding job with extensive family responsibilities, does not exercise outside of work, and is troubled by focal left LBP that she would like to be "fixed." As with all patients, it is important to ask about symptoms or historical features that would be suggestive of cancer or infection (such as fevers, weight loss, and prior cancer history) in the context of a comprehensive medical history. Questions about neurologic involvement such as weakness and incontinence are essential, as is a basic neurologic exam of the lower extremities. For all patients, it is also critical to inquire about mood changes (depression, anxiety, and fear in particular), stress at home or work, sleep, and diet. A history of trauma or marginalization, either socially or medically, is also important to understand in engaging with the patient's needs and experiences. Goals beyond pain reduction should routinely be explored. What does she like to do? What is she not doing? Does she have goals for the future that she wants to pursue? The answers to these questions are what drive rehabilitation and offer solutions to engage her in more effective exercise and self-care.

Assuming an otherwise benign medical history, no neurologic or "red flag" concerns, and no issues with anxiety, depression, or other significant stressors beyond what we know, the care of this patient revolves around reassurance, providing support to improve her situation, and engaging her in more effective self-care. Explaining that there is nothing to suggest anything particularly "bad" is occurring and that her X-rays are consistent with her age is a place to start. Treatment is directed toward making her better around whatever may be going on in her spine. Physical therapy would be helpful here to address range of motion, gait and movement patterns, trunk/abdominal function, work-specific tasks, and transitioning her to an independent exercise program to train her for her work. As an analogy, if she were a 48-year-old tennis player, she might have to stretch, walk, and do some resistance training to keep her body prepared for tennis. As she has a very physical job, she has to train for the demands of that. The job alone does not help with this, as tennis alone does not help the tennis player. Helping her explore her interests and available resources for exercise, like a community center, pool, fitness classes, online resources, or a home exercise space, and helping her think through barriers to exercise and self-care, which can be significant as a single parent with a full-time job, can be helpful. It may well be that she does not see how she can effectively take care of herself rather than that she does not want to.

There is no indication for further imaging in this patient. Over-the-counter analgesics are appropriate. There is no role here for opiates, muscle relaxants, or other sedating medications. There is no indication for any interventional procedure. A soft brace or corset could be considered for her work. These essentially act as postural reminders more than structural stabilizers and can be useful situationally. They should not be worn continuously. Advice to stretch, get off her feet, work with her physical therapist, and use topical heat periodically can all be helpful. Compassion, articulating an understanding of her stresses and fears, validating her desire to eliminate the source of her pain while explaining our limitations in doing so, and helping her create a more desired state to pursue through rehabilitation, exercise, and better health can all go a long way toward improving her current situation.

KEY POINTS

1. X-rays in adults commonly show age-related degenerative changes which have no association with LBP.
2. Specific treatments to "fix" the spine are elusive, and treatment should be directed more toward function.
3. Improving self-care and directing exercise toward work or activity-specific functional tasks are helpful approaches to management.
4. For the overwhelming majority of patients, there is no substantial evidence that medical or surgical interventions can "fix" LBP. This should not be the goal of care.

Further reading

1. Kalichman L, Kim DH, Li L, Guermazi A, Hunter DJ. Computed tomography-evaluated features of spinal degeneration: prevalence, intercorrelation, and association with self-reported low back pain. Spine J. 2010 Mar;10(3):200–208. doi: 10.1016/j.spinee.2009.10.018. Epub 2009 Dec 16. PMID: 20006557; PMCID: PMC3686273.
2. Maas ET, Ostelo RW, Niemisto L, Jousimaa J, et al. Radiofrequency denervation for chronic low back pain. Cochrane Database Syst Rev. 2015 Oct 23;2015(10):CD008572. doi: 10.1002/14651858.CD008572.pub2. PMID: 26495910; PMCID: PMC8782593.
3. Malik KM, Cohen SP, Walega DR, Benzon HT. Diagnostic criteria and treatment of discogenic pain: a systematic review of recent clinical literature. Spine J. 2013 Nov;13(11):1675–1689. doi: 10.1016/j.spinee.2013.06.063. Epub 2013 Aug 28. PMID: 23993035.

4 "Of Course My Back Hurts— I Have Two Bulging Discs"

Charles Davis, Christopher J. Standaert, Jeffrey G. Jarvik

When you ask how you can help them today, your new 52-year-old patient replies, "I have two bulging discs." They go on to complain of ongoing axial low back pain (LBP) without radiating leg pain, noting that a previous provider obtained a lumbar magnetic resonance imaging (MRI) study last year that revealed the disc issues. They add that they can "feel" the disc bulges in their back. You ultimately suggest exercise, over-the-counter analgesics, and offer a referral to physical therapy. The patient asks how those things will "fix" their discs and if they have "degenerative disc disease" (DDD). They note family members are severely limited by that condition and your patient does not want to "end up like them."

What do you do now?

Although spinal imaging can be very helpful in identifying spinal pathology, very few spines actually appear "normal" on MRI, and the majority of "abnormalities" noted are generally quite common, age-related changes. Findings of "disc degeneration" are essentially ubiquitous as people age, and focal findings of disc bulging, disc desiccation, and disc herniations generally are not identifiable sources of LBP. Unfortunately, patients often perceive these findings as significant, if not catastrophic, in their attempts to understand their pain. It is critical that medical providers understand the nature and prevalence of imaging findings and that they can translate and interpret the findings appropriately for their patients. Anything deemed "abnormal" by a patient can be frightening. They typically do not have a basis for distinguishing changes that occur with normal human aging from those that are truly pathologic or sources of pain. Reinforcing a belief that a particular normal or unrelated finding is a cause of pain can be harmful to patients and can lead to unhealthy beliefs about disability or an excessive desire for a structural cure.

It is helpful to understand normal disc anatomy, normal changes that occur during life, and radiologic terminology. This can all make it easier to interpret diagnostic imaging reports. As its name implies, an intervertebral disc is situated between two roughly cylindrical vertebral bodies. There is a ligamentous periphery called the anulus fibrosus with concentric layers of collagen fibers that alternate directions, providing excellent support for axial loads but perhaps leaving the disc more vulnerable to focal shear forces. The center of the disc is the gelatinous nucleus pulposus. In the idealized state, discs are uniform in height and with a typically well-hydrated nucleus (around 80% water), which allows both motion and the ability to withstand compressive loads. The vertebral endplate is a specialized portion of the vertebral body that is at the interface of the disc and the vertebral body. It allows for diffusion of water and solutes and serves as an anchoring point for the collagen fibers in the disc.

As part of normal human growth and aging, the discs and endplates undergo expected changes that are seen on MRI as early as adolescence. A common occurrence is an increase in collagen fibers in the nucleus, which contributes to a relative loss of water content. This is reflected as relatively dark signal on T2-weighted images on MRI, a finding that may be reported as disc desiccation or disc signal loss, and is sometimes called a "black disc,"

TABLE 4.1 **Estimated age-specific rates of imaging findings in people without LBP**

Imaging finding	Age (years)						
	20	30	40	50	60	70	80
Disc degeneration	37%	52%	68%	80%	88%	93%	96%
Disc height loss	24%	34%	45%	56%	67%	76%	84%
Disc bulge	30%	40%	50%	60%	69%	77%	84%
Disc protrusion	29%	31%	33%	36%	38%	40%	43%
Annular fissure	19%	20%	22%	23%	25%	27%	29%
Facet degeneration	4%	9%	18%	32%	50%	69%	83%
Spondylolisthesis	3%	5%	8%	14%	23%	35%	50%

Modified from Brinjikji W, Luetmer PH, Comstock B, et al. Systematic literature review of imaging features of spinal degeneration in asymptomatic populations. Am J Neuroradiol. 2015;36(4):811–816. doi:10.3174/ajnr.A4173.

a term that should be avoided due to false negative connotations of the language. An annular fissure is seen as a thin bright line within the annulus fibrosis on T2-weighted images. Although commonly called an "annular tear," this term is not accurate (and also should be avoided) as it implies an association with trauma. In studies of people without LBP, annular fissures are seen in 20–30% of adults of all ages, and they are generally not causally related to LBP.

Disc bulging and disc herniations are also commonly seen in those without LBP and increase in frequency with age (see Table 4.1). In the idealized state, the boundaries of an intervertebral disc align with the boundaries of the adjacent vertebral bodies. Disc bulges and herniations refer to an extension of the wall of or portion of a disc beyond the normal boundaries of the bone (see Figure 4.1). If the region of disc material extending beyond the normal borders of the vertebrae is more than 25% of the disc circumference, it is called a disc bulge. If a more focal portion of the disc (up to 25% of its circumference) extends beyond the normal borders of the vertebrae, it is called a disc herniation. A disc herniation is further classified as: a protrusion if it is wider at its base than it is at its outer tip (the shape of a bell

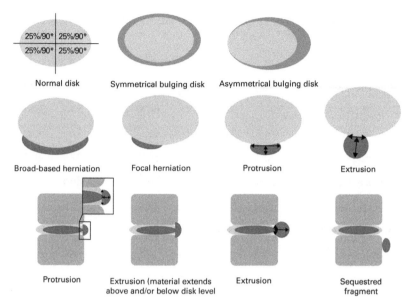

25%/90* | 25%/90*
25%/90* | 25%/90*

Normal disk   Symmetrical bulging disk   Asymmetrical bulging disk

Broad-based herniation   Focal herniation   Protrusion   Extrusion

Protrusion   Extrusion (material extends above and/or below disk level   Extrusion   Sequestred fragment

FIGURE 4.1. Disc bulge and disc herniation morphology.

From: Waldt S, Gersing A, Brügel M. Measurements and classifications in spine imaging. Semin Musculoskelet Radiol. 2014 Jul;18(3):219–227. doi: 10.1055/s-0034-1375565. Epub 2014 Jun 4.

curve); an extrusion if it is narrower at its base than at its outside edge (the shape of a mushroom); or a sequestration (or free fragment) if the extruded disc material separates from the main body of the disc.

Disc extrusions and sequestrations are relatively infrequent in the population and are more clearly related to radicular pain than other forms of herniation. These two subtypes of herniations also have extremely high rates of spontaneous regression on serial imaging, with almost half of sequestrations resolving entirely over time. Given that one-third of asymptomatic individuals will have a disc herniation by age 40, any correlation between the presence of a disc herniation and radicular pain needs to be made with a full understanding of a patient's clinical presentation. It is very difficult, if not impossible, to correlate a given disc bulge or disc herniation to axial LBP. Disc bulges are found on MRIs in the majority of people over 40 years old, but only a small minority of people over 40 have ongoing, disabling LBP. The two are generally not related.

The radiological term "disc degeneration" can be used when one or more of the above findings are present. This term does not indicate the presence of a disease process, which would be pathological, but rather the sequelae of normal aging. In fact, calling an imaging finding "degenerative disc disease," can be highly problematic as seen in the case presented above. This term is not well-defined or used in any specific way in either the medical literature or clinical practice, and aging is not a disease. More importantly, it medicalizes changes in the spine that are simply part of normal aging, and the words can be frightening for patients. It would be best for everyone to avoid the term "degenerative disc disease" altogether.

Beyond the disc, multiple other structural issues in the spine are frequently described in imaging reports. The vertebrae articulate posteriorly in the zygapophyseal or facet joints. Like other joints in the body, these have articular cartilage, joint fluid, and capsules. With age, changes seen on MRI include joint space narrowing, loss of cartilage, and osteophyte formation—a combination called facet degeneration or facet joint arthropathy. These findings are also extremely common and increase in prevalence with age (see Table 4.1). Spondylolisthesis (discussed in detail in chapters 8 and 9), scoliosis (chapter 10), and diffuse idiopathic skeletal hyperostosis (DISH) also increase in prevalence with age. These can be problematic or relevant in finite circumstances but are also not necessarily associated with LBP.

In other orthopedic conditions, imaging findings can be clearly associated with pathology and pain, such as a broken tibia. For LBP, a different mental framework is needed. The patient in the scenario above has had axial LBP (meaning that it is localized to the back and does not radiate to the buttocks or legs) for longer than 12 weeks, making it chronic in duration. This patient does not have any "red flag" signs or symptoms to suggest infection, malignancy, or a vertebral fracture. In accordance with treatment guidelines, you have suggested conservative measures without repeat imaging. After validating the patient's concerns about their family members' struggles with possible "degenerative disc disease," it is best to redirect their attention away from their focus on the structural issues identified on their imaging. Explain to the patient that if you were to pull ten 52-year-old people without LBP into your office and put them in an MRI machine, the MRIs would show that six of those 10 also have bulging discs. You can also explain that "degenerative disc disease" is not really a disease at all and does not mean that their spine will deteriorate. An adage in radiology is "don't treat the image, treat the patient." This is especially true for back pain since there is almost always a finding on imaging that one could think of treating. Unfortunately, it is difficult, if not impossible, to know if that finding is the culprit.

Although it seems logical that the severity of MRI findings would help to predict the success of conservative therapy, systematic reviews have not found a consistent association between the two. When it comes to the spinal MRI findings mentioned above, no such relationship exists. This patient is worried about a progressive loss of functionality, and you can assure them that there is no evidence that a bulging disc predicts a decline in function. Moreover, the exercises and physical therapy that you have prescribed are likely to help their function and are evidence-based.

There have been a number of studies exploring how social determinants of health relate to chronic LBP. Among many relationships detected, the strongest associations are with low socioeconomic status and low educational attainment. These findings fit with population health's known social gradient—that there is a proportional relationship between a person's health status and socioeconomic position. Given the complex biopsychosocial construct of chronic LBP, clinicians need to be aware of mental health, social, and financial challenges, or threats that their patients may face, and it would be judicious of future LBP studies to explore these relationships in conjunction with imaging findings.

There are a number of evidence-based guidelines for the diagnosis and treatment of LBP published by reputable groups, such as the American College of Physicians. One recent review found that by simply following these clinical guidelines, Medicare costs could be reduced by $362 million each year. While it has been shown that patient expectations often drive the escalation toward early MRI or other imaging for LBP, the strong evidence against early advanced diagnostic imaging has led government organizations and medical societies to recommend against any lumbar spine imaging for the first four to six weeks following initial presentation as long as there are no "red flags." Early imaging for LBP has been associated with higher rates of surgery, higher costs, and worse clinical outcomes. Of course, sometimes buried in the haystack of age-related, degenerative findings on imaging, there may an occasional "needle," but identifying this takes a full understanding of the imaging, the pathology, and the clinical state of the patient. Generally, these are the less common or "outlier" type findings. Clinicians must proceed cautiously and always be skeptical about identifying an imaging finding as the cause of a patient's back pain.

KEY POINTS

1. Findings of disc degeneration are a normal manifestation of aging and are commonly seen on spinal imaging in people without LBP.
2. "Degenerative disc disease" is an inaccurate and poorly defined phrase that is associated with harmful effects on patients. It should not be used.
3. Disc bulges and disc herniations are present in 50% and 33% of the population, respectively, by age 40. Medical providers need to be skeptical about any causal relationship they may have to a given patient's LBP.
4. Early spinal imaging in the absence of clear, acute medical/ neurological concerns has been associated with higher costs and worse clinical outcomes.
5. LBP needs to be viewed as a biopsychosocial process, and excessive "medicalization" of pain associated with imaging findings needs to be actively discouraged.

Further reading
1. Brinjikji W, Luetmer PH, Comstock B, et al. Systematic literature review of imaging features of spinal degeneration in asymptomatic populations. Am J Neuroradiol. 2015;36(4):811–816. doi:10.3174/ajnr.A4173.
2. Roudsari B, Jarvik JG. Lumbar spine MRI for low back pain: indications and yield. Am J Roentgenol. 2010;195(3):550–559. doi:10.2214/AJR.10.4367.
3. Qaseem A, Wilt TJ, McLean RM, Forciea MA. Noninvasive treatments for acute, subacute, and chronic low back pain: a clinical practice guideline from

the American College of Physicians. Ann Intern Med. 2017;166(7):514–530. doi:10.7326/M16-2367.

4. Fardon DF, Williams AL, Dohring EJ, Murtagh FR, Rothman SLG, Sze GK. Lumbar disc nomenclature: version 2.0: recommendations of the combined task forces of the North American Spine Society, the American Society of Spine Radiology, and the American Society of Neuroradiology. Spine. 2014;14(11):2525–2545. doi:10.1016/j.spinee.2014.04.022.

5. Jarvik JG, Gold LS, Comstock BA, et al. Association of early imaging for back pain with clinical outcomes in older adults. JAMA. 2015;313(11):1143–1153. doi:10.1001/jama.2015.1871.

6. Milani CJ, Rundell S, Jarvik JG, et al. Associations of race and ethnicity with patient-reported outcomes and health care utilization among older adults initiating a new episode of care for back pain. Spine. 2018 Jul 15;43(14):1007–1017.

5 "It's My Sciatica.": Radiating Leg Pain in a 37-Year-Old

William Taylor Riden, Christopher J. Standaert, Kevin A. Carneiro

A 37-year-old female presents with 3 weeks of low back pain (LBP) with "sciatica" and numbness in her left leg. The pain started when she was putting on her shoes one morning. There was no other injury. She cannot sit for more than 15 minutes without experiencing pain in her leg but feels better standing. Sleep is difficult. It is hard to get out of the house in the morning due to her pain. She works in an office and struggles with sitting at the computer long enough to work effectively. The pain runs from her low back into her posterior calf. She feels pins and needles in the sole of her foot at times but does not feel weak or have any changes in bowel or bladder function. She is healthy otherwise and takes no prescription medications. She has been taking over the counter analgesics with only minimal benefit.

What do you do now?

The presence of leg pain or neurologic concerns with LBP represents a different clinical situation than LBP alone. Leg pain arising from the lumbar spine is generally related to a problem affecting the lumbar nerve root. The specific presentation above is suggestive of a posterolateral disc herniation affecting the S1 nerve root. Lumbar disc herniations are a common clinical problem most often affecting those in their 30s or 40s. When symptomatic, they are often associated with LBP and pain radiating down one or both legs depending on the location of the herniation. As acute disc herniations largely improve with time, they are most commonly treated with symptom management, reassurance, patient education about how to recognize progressive or concerning neurologic symptoms, encouragement to maintain (and gradually progress) activity within tolerance, and patience.

Lumbar radicular pain has an estimated prevalence of 9.8 cases per 1000 people. While "radiculitis" refers to inflammation affecting a nerve root, "radiculopathy" is defined as spinal nerve root dysfunction causing dermatomal pain and paresthesia, myotomal weakness, and/or impaired deep tendon reflexes. "Sciatica" as a symptom is nonspecific and simply refers to pain radiating from the low back down the leg. Of those who present with lumbar radicular pain, it is generally reported that symptoms will subside in about 90% of patients, typically within 6–12 weeks, with conservative treatment.

Physiologically, lumbar discs are involved with transmitting loads and providing flexibility to facilitate movement. The structure of the disc includes the outer annulus fibrosus and inner nucleus pulposus. Theoretically, a disc herniation is related to a tear in the annulus through with a portion of the nucleus can protrude. This is defined radiographically by a focal extension of disc material (representing 25% or less of the total circumference of the disc, see chapter 4) beyond the normal confines of the annulus. About 95% of lumbar disc herniations occur at the L4/5 and L5/S1 levels, likely related to the high degree of motion and physiologic load at these levels. Most of these occur in the posterolateral portion of the disc, just off midline but within the spinal canal (see Figure 5.1). When studied with serial spinal imaging, about two-thirds of those sustaining an acute disc herniation show regression/healing of the disc within 12 months.

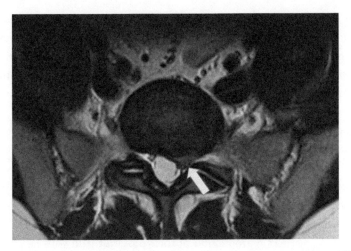

FIGURE 5.1. Axial T2 MRI images MRI showing posterolateral lumbar disc herniation at L5/S1 on the left, displacing the left S1 nerve root (see arrow).

When patients present to clinic with low back and leg pain, it is important to characterize the symptoms in a stepwise fashion. In this case, we know the patient had an acute onset of pain after putting on her shoes. This is a rather ordinary activity that may or may not have any actual connection to the disc herniating. Although people often associate their disc injury to whatever they were doing around the onset of their pain, disc herniations are largely random events. This patient describes worsening pain with flexion and bending forward, which can suggest pain arising from a disc. Increased pain with lifting, coughing, sneezing, or Valsalva are also typically seen in a disc herniation. This patient's pain is worse with sitting and lying flat and better with standing, further supporting a disc process as the source of her pain. She describes the pain in her leg as "pins and needles," implying a neuropathic (nerve) process.

Physical examination should include an assessment of vital signs and overall appearance of the patient in the exam room. When focusing on the lumbosacral spine, we use a systematic approach including inspection, palpation, range of motion, strength, sensation, special tests, and gait assessment. We start with inspection looking for any asymmetry in musculature, previous site of surgical incisions, rashes, erythema, or swelling. We then move to palpation of the spinous processes, paraspinal muscles, surrounding musculature in the gluteal region, sacrum, greater trochanters, and groin. Next, we assess range of motion in the lumbosacral spine in flexion and extension (always within what is comfortable for the patient), primarily looking for motion that may reproduce their symptoms or be otherwise restricted. A thorough neurologic exam is required to assess strength, sensation, and reflexes. Gait testing should include heel and toe walking to assess dorsiflexion and plantarflexion strength. Provocative maneuvers suggesting a nerve root process, like a straight leg raise test, can be performed. The straight leg raise test is intended to put tension on the L5 and S1 nerve roots and is done by slowly elevating the leg (with the knee straight) while the patient is laying supine. This test is positive if the patient experiences reproduction of their posterior pain with elevation of the leg at 30–60 degrees (measured at the hip). This and similar tests have limited sensitivity and specificity and are more additive to the clinical picture than diagnostic.

In patients who continue to have low back and leg pain beyond six weeks or in those with severe pain or neurological loss, it is reasonable to consider diagnostic imaging. X-rays are an appropriate step in those with persisting symptoms and should always be obtained if there are concerns for red flag conditions including fracture, tumor, infection, or cauda equina syndrome. In those with severe or persisting radicular pain and/or neurological loss, advanced imaging, such as a magnetic resonance imaging (MRI), can be helpful, with the caveat that about one-third of asymptomatic adults have disc herniations on MRI (see chapter 4). It is critically important to correlate any findings on imaging with the medical history, findings on physical examination, and other diagnostic studies to draw any potential causal connections between what is found on imaging and a given patient's problem. Just because a disc herniation is identified in an MRI report does not mean that it is a problem. In general, MRI or other advanced imaging is required before considering surgery or other interventional care.

As discussed earlier, it is reported that approximately 90% of patients will experience improvement in symptoms with nonsurgical treatments alone. In the absence of red flag signs, the most recent guidelines from the American College of Physicians emphasize non-pharmacological medical treatment for LBP. Common available nonsurgical treatments include relative rest with activity modification, superficial heat, massage, acupuncture, spinal manipulation, and physical therapy. There are little data as to the efficacy of any of these specifically in the setting of radicular pain and/or a disc herniation. Nonsteroidal anti-inflammatory drugs (NSAIDs) and muscle relaxants can be used initially. There is debate regarding the use of oral steroids in patients with radicular pain. In general, in patients with symptoms less than 3 months, oral steroids have shown benefit in improving function but not pain. Encouraging gentle, low impact activity, like walking or swimming, and efforts at pain reduction with the above treatments can be used to facilitate recovery. The goal of early treatment is to maintain basic function and activity within tolerance while allowing time for recovery.

If pain persists after several months, providers can consider additional medications including gabapentin, pregabalin, tricyclic antidepressants (TCA), and serotonin and norepinephrine reuptake inhibitors (SNRI), although there are no substantial data supporting the use of any of these specifically for persistent radicular pain. For patients with persistent pain, we assess for psychosocial factors that could be contributing to their pain, distress, or disability. We also counsel patients on lifestyle modifications including weight loss, aerobic exercise, ergonomics, sleep hygiene, and nutrition. Epidural steroid injections can be included in the treatment plan for a patient with a lumbar disc herniation with radiculopathy. There is evidence that epidural steroid injections can improve radicular pain associated with a disc herniation in the short term (weeks). However, benefits and risks must be considered, given costs and potential adverse effects of corticosteroid injections.

There is a potential role for surgery for those with a disc herniation resulting in ongoing (greater than 6–12 weeks), severe and limiting radicular pain, or significant or progressive weakness. Those with acutely progressive weakness should consult with a spine surgeon urgently, as they are at risk for worsening motor deficits that could result in long-term functional impairments. Typically, for a one level disc herniation, the surgical treatment of choice is a microdiscectomy. In the United States, surgery is performed in about 10–15% of patients with a lumbar disc herniation and radiculopathy with the vast majority achieving sustained improvement in pain. However, about 10% of those undergoing a microdiscectomy experience a perioperative complication, and about 7% will require another spine surgery within 1 year.

For the patient presented above, we would obtain an expanded history and perform a careful neurologic exam. Physical examination should include heel and toe walking, which assess the L5 and S1 nerve roots, respectively. Here we are concerned for an S1 radiculopathy as her pain and numbness follow the S1 dermatome. Plantar flexion is the dominant motor function controlled by the S1 root, which is hard to assess well by applying manual resistance. It is better to assess toe walking and the ability to do single-leg toe raises. The latter are performed by standing on one leg and rising up on the toes of that leg, generally with an adjacent countertop or similar item for support. A young to middle-aged adult with normal strength should be able to do this 10 times. Deep tendon reflexes of the Achilles tendon ("ankle-jerks") are also important to test as a loss (or relative reduction) of this reflex on one side would be consistent with an S1 nerve root process on that side. In this case, the patient's history reveals no red flag concerns, and her neurological examination is normal, although she has a mildly positive straight leg raise test on the left.

We can tell her that her examination is re-assuring and that there is no need for urgent imaging, surgery, or similar care. It is possible that she has sustained a disc herniation. If so, she is highly likely to improve over the next 6–12 weeks, although full recovery may take 6–12 months. We could consider oral steroids, NSAIDs, and/or a muscle relaxant to assist with pain or sleep. NSIADs generally have the fewest side effects or risks of these options, so they may be a preferrable first step. Patient is initially encouraged to walk and activity as tolerated. If pain doesn't resolve on it's own in 2–4 weeks, engaging in a formal physical therapy program and medication adjustments could be considered. Axial imaging (e.g. MRI) would be considered if patient is not continuing to improve or develops a neurologic deficit. From there, an ESI could be considered for relief of radicular pain (although this is not expected to improve neurological loss or LBP). Surgical consultation should be obtained urgently if she develops progressive weakness but could also be considered if her pain is limiting her function and persists after at least 6–12 weeks, and there is no improvement with nonsurgical measures and time.

KEY POINTS

1. Lumbar disc herniations generally occur without a specific precipitating event.
2. The majority of lumbar disc herniations (~95%) occur at the L4/L5, L5/S1 levels.
3. The vast majority of patients with lumbar disc herniation and radiculopathy will improve within 6–12 weeks with symptom management and nonoperative care.
4. Approximately 90% of those with a symptomatic lumbar disc herniation can be successfully managed without surgery.
5. A thorough physical examination is important, paying close attention to suspected nerve roots involved.

Further reading
1. Casey E. Natural history of radiculopathy. Phys Med Rehabil Clin N Am. 2011 Feb;22(1):1–5. doi: 10.1016/j.pmr.2010.10.001. Epub 2010 Dec 3. PMID: 21292142.
2. Delgado-López PD, Rodríguez-Salazar A, Martín-Alonso J, Martín-Velasco V. [Lumbar disc herniation: Natural history, role of physical examination, timing of surgery, treatment options and conflicts of interests]. Neurocirugia (Astur). 2017 May-Jun;28(3):124–134. Spanish. doi: 10.1016/j.neucir.2016.11.004. Epub 2017 Jan 25. PMID: 28130015.
3. Goldberg H, Firtch W, Tyburski M, et al. Oral steroids for acute radiculopathy due to a herniated lumbar disk: a randomized clinical trial. JAMA. 2015 May 19;313(19):1915–1923. doi: 10.1001/jama.2015.4468. PMID: 25988461; PMCID: PMC5875432.
4. Qaseem A, Wilt TJ, McLean RM, Forciea MA; Clinical Guidelines Committee of the American College of Physicians. Noninvasive treatments for acute, subacute, and chronic low back pain: a clinical practice guideline from the American College of Physicians. Ann Intern Med. 2017 Apr 4;166(7):514–530. doi: 10.7326/M16-2367. Epub 2017 Feb 14. PMID: 28192789.
5. Annaswamy TM, Taylor C. Lumbar disc disorders. PM&R Knowledge Now. 2017 https://now.aapmr.org/lumbar-disc-disorders/.

6 "I Can't Stand Up!": Severe Acute Pain in a 63-Year-Old Male

Eman Kazi, Christopher J. Standaert

A long-established patient presents with acute, severe pain into his left thigh. He is 63, you have known him for years, and he has never had this kind of pain before. There was no injury that he could identify. He notes some pain in his right low back or flank but gets severe pain into the front of his right thigh whenever he tries to stand up straight. He has some discomfort sitting in your exam room but is unable to stand up straight due to pain extending down his right thigh to the knee. There is no calf pain. He has no fever or dysuria. He has stable hypertension and dyslipidemia and is taking hydrochlorothiazide and a statin medication. He appears remarkably uncomfortable with attempts at walking and tends to remain flexed forward at the waist when doing so.

What do you do now?

This patient clearly presents with an acute, markedly painful condition. Given the distribution of pain, one has to consider renal issues such as a kidney stone or an acute problem with the hip joint, both of which are frequently pursued in this presentation before the correct diagnosis is made. Although problems with both the hip and renal system can refer pain down the front of the thigh, this can also arise from the L2, L3, or L4 nerve roots. Pain from these roots follows a pattern distinctly different than pain from L5 and S1, which are more commonly affected and typically associated with pain and/or numbness radiating down the posterolateral leg to the calf or foot. Generally speaking, L2 refers to the upper anterior thigh, L3 to the mid to lower anterior thigh or knee, and L4 to the knee region down into the anterior to medial calf. The distribution of pain in the patient presented is most typical of L3, and this presentation is relatively distinct for what is termed a "far lateral disc herniation," affecting the L3 root just after it has passed through the neural foramen. This needs to be recognized as a unique pathologic and clinical entity with characteristics that distinguish it from other disc issues. It is critical to work through the clinical and diagnostic evaluation of these patients to avoid common misdiagnoses and incorrect treatment.

Disc herniations are a relatively common injury, affecting up to 2% of adults annually. They occur in men more than women at almost a 2:1 ratio, most commonly in individuals between 30 and 50 years old. Despite the potential to cause severe pain, motor weakness, or cauda equina compression, the vast majority of disc herniations are managed nonoperatively, with about 10% of patients being treated surgically. Of clinically relevant disc herniations, 95% occur at L4/5 or L5/S1. These will classically present with "sciatica" (meaning pain that travels from the back, down the leg, and extending past the knee) in conjunction with a range of other findings, including numbness in the foot and/or toes and weakness in leg musculature that can result in a foot drop (dorsiflexion—the L5 root) or trouble raising up onto the toes (plantar flexion—the S1 root). Patients will often present with severe back and/or leg pain and appear very uncomfortable. This can be a concerning presentation, and all of these patients need to be screened for "red flags" (suggestive of tumor, fracture, infection, or severe neurological injury) and undergo an appropriate physical examination. The pain distribution from a disc herniation can overlap with a variety of etiologies including spine, hip, soft tissues in the leg, peripheral nerve, vasculature, or renal. For these reasons, diagnosis and treatment can be challenging, and patients must be investigated thoroughly.

As noted, a unique subset of lumbar disc herniations are termed "far lateral" disc herniations. This term refers to the location of the disc relative to the spinal canal. A lumbar disc has two main components: the outer annulus fibrosis, a containing/structural wall composed of overlapping layers of collagen fibers, and the nucleus pulposus, the more gelatinous/hydrated center of the disc. In an idealized disc herniation, the annulus fibrosis tears or fails in a focal region, allowing a portion of the nucleus to herniate out through the opening (disc pathology and terminology is discussed further in chapter 4). Most commonly, disc herniations occur posterolaterally, meaning just lateral to the middle of the posterior aspect of the disc inside the spinal canal, roughly at the 5:00 and 7:00 positions if looking at an axial magnetic resonance imaging (MRI) or computed tomography (CT) image (Figure 6.1, see chapter 5 for a discussion of posterolateral disc herniations). If a nerve root is affected by a disc in this location, it is most commonly the descending root that has exited from the dura but not from the spinal canal yet. A posterolateral L3/L4 disc herniation would therefore affect the L4 root and an L4/L5 posterolateral disc herniation would affect the L5 root. In a far lateral disc herniation, the annular disruption and disc herniation occur outside of the spinal canal, at roughly the 3:00–4:00 or

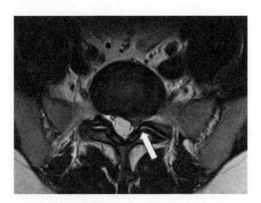

FIGURE 6.1. Axial T2 weighted MRI image showing a left posterolateral disc herniation (see arrow). Note that this is within the spinal canal.

8:00–9:00 positions if looking at an axial MRI or CT image (Figure 6.2). These disc fragments affect the nerve root that has already left the spinal canal at that level. Thus, a far lateral disc herniation at L3/L4 would affect the L3 root, and a far lateral disc herniation at L4/L5 would affect the L4 root. Importantly, the dorsal root ganglia, comprised of the cell bodies of the sensory neurons of the nerve root, is located in the nerve root lateral to the foramen and can be directly affected by a far lateral disc herniation, potentially accounting for the distinctly painful presentation associated with these disc herniations.

Far lateral disc herniations comprise 1–10% of disc herniations, but they are a unique clinical syndrome and should be approached as such. There are a number of clinical and demographic features that distinguish those with a far lateral disc herniation from those with a posterolateral herniation. Those with a far lateral disc tend to be older, typically 50 to 80 years old, and they tend to be distributed evenly between males and females. Far lateral disc herniations tend to occur higher in the spine, affecting the L3 and L4 roots most commonly. They also are associated with more severe leg pain and higher rates of sensory dysesthesia and motor weakness than posterolateral disc herniations. Given the location of far lateral disc herniations, pain tends to refer into the hip, anterior thigh, and/or anterior calf. Importantly, the pain is usually far worse with standing than sitting, a

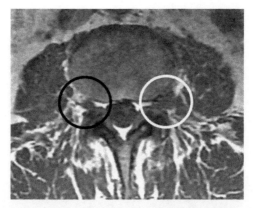

FIGURE 6.2. Axial T1 weighted MRI image with a left far lateral disc herniation. The white circle surrounds the disc herniation, seen as a dark oval shape, outside of the spinal canal. Contrast this with the normal nerve root on the other side, which is surrounded by the black circle.

pattern very different from the majority of those with a posterolateral disc herniation (who tend to have more pain sitting and relief with standing). As a snapshot, patients with acute far lateral disc herniations are generally over 50, come into the exam room flexed forward, are unable to stand erect without severe leg pain, and have neurologic abnormalities on exam.

Patients presenting to clinic with pain from a far lateral disc herniation can easily be misdiagnosed. Clinicians will need to conduct a focused physical exam to recognize a far lateral disc herniation and separate it from other possible diagnoses. The differential diagnosis can include nephrolithiasis, hip osteoarthritis, a psoas hemorrhage (often associated with anticoagulants), a diabetic lumbosacral radiculoplexus neuropathy (diabetic amyotrophy), or a pathologic fracture. Neurologic examination is *key* to diagnosing a far lateral disc herniation. Unlike patients with pain originating in the hip or renal systems, patients with far lateral disc herniations will often exhibit loss of the patellar reflex, weakness in hip flexion and/or knee extension, and loss of sensation in the anterior to medial thigh or the anterior to medial calf. They tend to have pain with spinal extension but not with hip motion independent of this. The pain is generally reduced when sitting.

The diagnostic evaluation may require several studies. An X-ray of the hip joint can rule out most hip pathology, although hip osteoarthritis is not an uncommon asymptomatic finding in this age group. Renal evaluation can be pursued if nephrolithiasis is highly suspected, but this would not be associated with neurologic deficits. X-rays of the lumbar spine with flexion/extension views should be obtained to assess for scoliosis, spondylolisthesis, or other bone pathology. MRI is the test of choice to identify a far lateral disc herniation (Figure 6.2). As these herniations are uncommon, they can be missed by those reading the images, particularly if they are not directed to do so by the ordering physician. If there is a high degree of suspicion for a far lateral disc herniation in the upper lumbar spine, a specific review of the MRI for this entity should be done. Electrodiagnostic testing could potentially help in distinguishing a radiculopathy from a plexopathy, a radiculoplexus neuropathy, or a femoral mononeuropathy. This would typically not be needed for a clearly identified far lateral disc herniation that correlates with the clinical presentation.

Data specifically related to the treatment of far lateral disc herniations are sparse. As with other disc herniations, most patients seem to improve spontaneously over weeks to months, and conservative treatment is the preferred initial approach. Pain management with over the counter analgesics is appropriate. If those are ineffective, oral steroids or an epidural steroid injection may be considered. Recent evidence has shown that gabapentinoids are generally not useful in spinal pain, although there is some evidence of benefit from duloxetine. Keeping patients active and moving within their pain tolerance is important; opiates should generally be avoided in spinal pain and always used with caution and in a time-limited fashion when prescribed. Surgery is an appropriate consideration for some patients. As with other disc herniations, this is performed in a minority of patients, given that most will have substantial resolution of symptoms over time without surgical intervention. Surgical approaches for far lateral disc herniations vary and are distinct from a more common micro-discectomy for a posterolateral disc herniation. However, outcomes on the whole seem to be similar for patients undergoing surgery for either a far lateral or a posterolateral disc herniation.

The patient described above presents with acute, severe left thigh pain and a history suggestive of a far lateral disc herniation. He should certainly be questioned about red flag symptoms like neurologic loss, fever, and trauma and, in this case, diabetes, hematuria or a history of renal issues. Exam should include motor and sensory testing and examination of lower extremity reflexes. His hip should be evaluated for pain with range of motion and his back for tenderness, range of motion (within pain tolerance), or other abnormalities. A reduced patellar reflex, weakness of hip flexion, and sensory loss in the distal medial thigh on the right would all be consistent with an L3 radiculopathy. It would be appropriate to obtain X-rays of his hip and lumbar spine. Given the differential diagnosis for these patients, an MRI to confirm the presence of a disc herniation that correlates with identified neurologic abnormalities is helpful. He has severe pain, warranting some form of analgesia ranging from over the counter medications to prescription NSAID's to either oral or epidural steroids or, rarely, a short course of opiates. All of these should be considered in the context of his medical situation and risk profile. If he has severe motor loss, progressive weakness, or severe pain despite time and nonoperative measures, surgical referral is appropriate. Physical therapy, focusing on restoring range of motion, leg strength, postural musculature, and function is highly appropriate for this patient. Light aerobic activity on a recumbent bike or water walking can be suggested early in order to keep the patient moving. In general, most patients will improve over time with conservative measures.

KEY POINTS

1. An upper lumbar radiculopathy is frequently misdiagnosed and needs to be considered in patients with acute flank and hip or thigh pain.
2. A thorough neurologic exam should be performed, focusing on proximal leg strength, sensation, and patellar reflex.
3. Patients with a far lateral disc herniation tend to be over 50 years old and have severe pain into their anterior thigh, as opposed to those with a posterolateral disc herniation who tend to be under 50 years old and have pain down the posterior to lateral thigh and calf.
4. MRI of the lumbar spine is the best imaging modality for identifying a far lateral disc herniation.
5. The vast majority of patients with a far lateral disc herniation and radiculopathy can be treated successfully with time and nonoperative care.

Further reading
1. Epstein NE. Foraminal and far lateral lumbar disc herniations: surgical alternatives and outcome measures. Spinal Cord. 2002 Oct;40(10):491–500. doi: 10.1038/sj.sc.3101319. PMID: 12235530.
2. Khan JM, McKinney D, Basques BA, et al. Clinical presentation and outcomes of patients with a lumbar far lateral herniated nucleus pulposus as compared to those with a central or paracentral herniation. Global Spine J. 2019 Aug;9(5):480–486. doi: 10.1177/2192568218800055. Epub 2018 Nov 18. PMID: 31431869; PMCID: PMC6686375.
3. Mérot OA, Maugars YM, Berthelot JM. Similar outcome despite slight clinical differences between lumbar radiculopathy induced by lateral versus medial disc herniations in patients without previous foraminal stenosis: a prospective cohort study with 1-year follow-up. Spine J. 2014 Aug 1;14(8):1526–1531. doi: 10.1016/j.spinee.2013.09.020. Epub 2013 Oct 11. PMID: 24291407.

4. Park HW, Park KS, Park MS, Kim SM, Chung SY, Lee DS. The comparisons of surgical outcomes and clinical characteristics between the far lateral lumbar disc herniations and the paramedian lumbar disc herniations. Korean J Spine. 2013 Sep;10(3):155–159. doi: 10.14245/kjs.2013.10.3.155. Epub 2013 Sep 30. PMID: 24757478; PMCID: PMC3941755.
5. Rust MS, Olivero WC. Far-lateral disc herniations: the results of conservative management. J Spinal Disord. 1999 Apr;12(2):138–140. PMID: 10229528.

7 "My Legs Hurt When I Walk a Few Blocks.": Back and Leg Pain in a 67-Year-Old

Christopher J. Standaert, Eman Kazi, Michael J. Schneider

A 67-year-old male complains of progressive low back and leg pain over the past 2 years. He has no history of back issues previously and notes no trauma or injury associated with the onset of his symptoms. He first noted some intermittent cramping and then numbness into his legs on longer walks. Over time, he developed pain into his posterior thighs and lateral calves on both sides that now occurs if he walks several blocks or stands for 15–20 minutes. He has some low back pain, but this is less problematic than the leg pain. He has tried some over the counter medications which help slightly. Mostly, he notes he has just stopped walking as much and is more sedentary. His weight has increased 20 lbs. over the past 2 years. He stopped mowing his lawn and doing most of his yard work. He does not really exercise otherwise and has never found physical therapy too helpful for other minor musculoskeletal problems. He does not feel weak and has no change in bowel or bladder function.

Diagnostic and therapeutic considerations are clearly different in older patients. For patients over 50 years old, degenerative conditions become much more common and can affect the spine and peripheral joints. Comorbidities like vascular disease and diabetes are also more common in older patients. In those 65 and older who develop low back pain (LBP), pain and the related disability tend to persist long-term for the majority. Although the patient presented above has LBP, his dominant complaints are leg pain, paresthesia, and functional decline. The presence of lower extremity complaints changes the clinical approach to LBP in all patients, as clinicians need to consider that neurologic structures may be compromised. In older patients, lumbar spinal stenosis (LSS) with neurogenic claudication (leg pain, numbness, fatigue, or related symptoms) or radiculopathy becomes a dominant concern for those with symptoms such as these. Working through an appropriate differential diagnosis and recognizing the variables that can be associated with LSS are important in managing these patients. Although LSS is the most common indication for spine surgery in older patients in the United States, most patients affected with LSS can be managed nonoperatively.

Strictly speaking, spinal stenosis is an anatomical and radiographic term that refers to narrowing of the spinal canal. *Radiographic stenosis* should be differentiated from the *clinical syndrome* of LSS, which is characterized by a specific cluster of clinical signs and symptoms. Most commonly, older individuals present with degenerative spinal stenosis, meaning the canal is narrowed by a collection of degenerative or age-related changes such as ligamentous thickening, disc height loss with bulging of the anulus fibrosis, and/or hypertrophy of the facet joints. Together, these degenerative changes gradually occlude or narrow the spinal canal over time (Figures 7.1A and B). Often, these issues can be accompanied by a degenerative spondylolisthesis (see chapter 9) that further narrows the canal (and also influences clinical decision-making).

Other processes can also narrow the spinal canal and cause anatomical spinal stenosis, either acutely or gradually over time. Disc herniations, epidural hematomas, synovial cysts, or tumors can all cause spinal stenosis with symptoms that are very similar to those associated with degenerative LSS, albeit with a more acute presentation for things like a disc herniation or hematoma. A small percentage of the population also has a congenitally

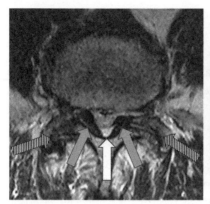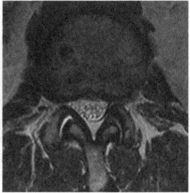

FIGURE 7.1. Axial T2 weighted MRI images. Figure 7.1A shows degenerative spinal canal stenosis at L4/L5 (white arrow) with ligamentum flavum hypertrophy (grey arrows) and facet arthropathy (stripped arrows). Figure 7.1B is from the L1/L2 level of the same person and shows minimal narrowing of the spinal canal with mild degenerative changes.

narrow spinal canal due to the structure of their vertebra. These individuals can present with symptoms suggestive of the clinical syndrome of LSS earlier in life related to minor structural issues that develop, given their congenitally limited space available at baseline. In the lumbar spine, LSS affects the cauda equina/nerve roots, resulting in radicular symptoms. In the cervical or thoracic spines (or above the distal end of the spinal cord which is typically around T12-L1), canal stenosis results in compression of the spinal cord with myelopathic symptoms or findings.

A normal adult lumbar spinal canal is about 12–18 mm across in anterior-posterior (AP) diameter. An AP diameter of less than 10 mm is generally considered "stenotic." Making a diagnosis of the clinical syndrome of LSS by imaging alone is problematic. On MRI studies of individuals without any low back symptoms, more than 10% of 40-year-olds have radiographic evidence of spinal stenosis in the lumbar spine. For patients over the age of 60 without any low back symptoms, 20–25% have radiographic LSS, generally resulting from common, natural degenerative changes that may not need treatment.

The degree of radiographic stenosis or anatomical narrowing is typically graded as "mild," "moderate," or "severe"; but in practice, these terms are poorly defined and variably applied by given individuals (including radiologists). There is no correlation between the severity of radiographic stenosis, the severity of symptoms, and the response to surgery or other treatments. Determining whether a patient's symptoms are related to any degree of stenosis identified on imaging and the appropriate treatment is really based on the clinical evaluation of the patient. This highlights the importance of differentiating between radiographic stenosis and the clinical syndrome of LSS.

The natural history of LSS is surprisingly understudied with limited populations monitored over time. There are no meaningful data available on any potential differential natural history by sex, ethnicity, or other factors. However, the limited data that has been published note a generally favorable history for those initially presenting without clear surgical indications. Of these individuals, the overwhelming majority are stable or even improve over time, with only a small percentage (10–15%) showing a clinical decline over 3 years.

The patient above clearly presents with a painful condition suggestive of degenerative LSS. However, several conditions may present in a similar manner or even overlap with the presentation of clinical LSS. The differential diagnosis can include peripheral vascular disease, peripheral polyneuropathy, and hip osteoarthritis. Peripheral vascular disease typically results in vascular claudication with lower extremity cramping, achiness, tightness, and fatigue in variable degrees, classically precipitated by walking a finite distance and relieved by standing or stopping (without sitting). A peripheral polyneuropathy can present with a range of symptoms including burning or paresthesia in the feet, numbness, loss of balance, gait changes, or weakness. These symptoms are not necessarily altered by position or activity, although the burning pain is commonly worse at night. Symptomatic hip osteoarthritis is most commonly associated with some combination of groin pain, anterior thigh pain, knee pain, difficulty ambulating, difficulty with getting into or out of a car, and relief with sitting. Posterior leg and hip/pelvic pain are less common (see Table 7.1).

Clinical LSS typically presents with neurogenic claudication, to be distinguished from vascular claudication. Symptoms of neurogenic claudication can include leg pain, cramping, heaviness, or fatigue with standing or walking, generally relieved by sitting or flexing forward at the waist (not just standing still). Often, these symptoms are separated from "neuroischemic"

TABLE 7.1 **Characteristics of Common Conditions Causing Lower Extremity Symptoms in Older Adults**

	Peripheral Vascular Disease	**Lumbar Spinal Stenosis**	**Hip Osteoarthritis**	**Peripheral Polyneuropathy**
Leg pain during walking	Yes (vascular claudication)	Yes (neurogenic claudication)	Yes	Not typical
Relief after resting	Yes, standing or sitting	Yes, only when sitting	Yes, with sitting or lying down	Not typical
Description of leg symptoms	Cramping, aching, tightness, fatigue	Tingling, numbness, heaviness, weakness, paresthesia	Deep ache, throbbing	Burning, tingling, or paresthesia in the feet
Relief with postural changes	No	Yes, with lumbar flexion	No	No
Relief using a shopping cart	No	Yes	Yes	No
Range of motion changes	No	Reduced lumbar spine extension	Reduced hip joint motion, particularly hip flexion, and internal rotation	No
Neurological changes on examination	No	Yes	No	Yes
Diagnostic confirmation	Ankle-brachial index Vascular doppler/ ultrasound	Lumbar MRI or CT myelogram, EMG/NCS	Plain X-ray of hips	EMG/NCS

Abbreviations: EMG/NCS, electromyography/nerve conduction studies.

symptoms like numbness, tingling, paresthesia, weakness, or loss of balance, again associated with standing or walking. The leg symptoms can be variable and often asymmetric. The cause of the symptoms in those with LSS is unclear but may be related to structural changes in the nerve roots resulting from chronic compression, impairment of microvascular flow, or impairment of venous flow. Similar mechanisms can result in neurological injury. There is less evidence that symptomatic degenerative LSS is an inflammatory process, likely explaining the general lack of benefit associated with the use of corticosteroids or similar anti-inflammatory medications.

Clinical evaluation should be utilized to screen for "red flag" conditions, distinguish between the various processes that can cause leg symptoms, assess the neurological status of the patient, and understand the functional and social implications of the presentation. Red flag conditions include fracture, tumor, infection, and severe or progressive neurological injury. Older patients are at higher risk of all of these. Trauma or acute onset of pain (even without trauma) might suggest a fracture, and tumor should be considered in anyone with a known history of cancer. Conditions associated with a peripheral neuropathy or vascular disease, such as diabetes or smoking, may be directly related to the presenting symptoms. Osteopenia or osteoporosis, prior cancer, obesity, prior orthopedic or spinal surgeries, and falls may influence diagnosis and management. Exercise history, recreational or vocational activities, care responsibilities, and a psychosocial history should be obtained for all patients. Depression, anxiety, and social isolation are common issues affecting both older individuals and those with chronic pain.

A history of leg symptoms in any combination of the above, especially numbness, tingling, and/or neurogenic claudication, that is initiated by standing or walking and relieved by sitting or flexing forward should raise suspicion of LSS. The "shopping cart sign," in which a patient's symptoms are relieved when walking with a shopping cart, is similarly suggestive of LSS.

Physical examination includes a direct examination of the spine looking for focal tenderness, scoliosis, and range of motion within comfort. Spinal extension often worsens or provokes the symptoms of spinal stenosis. Gait evaluation for weakness and balance deficits and testing for lower extremity strength, sensation, deep tendon reflexes, and Babinski reflexes should be performed. Weakness is concerning and may warrant surgical consultation. Soft touch, vibration/proprioception, and pin-prick sensation should all be tested. Diffuse distal sensory loss in a "stocking" pattern with loss of reflexes may indicate a peripheral polyneuropathy. Vibratory sensation loss is common in LSS and may increase the risk of falls. Upper motor neuron signs like a Babinski reflex or hyperreflexia are suggestive of a spinal cord or other central nervous system process and warrant evaluation beyond the lumbar spine, including a consideration for degenerative cervical myelopathy due to cervical spinal stenosis. Hip range of motion should also be assessed to rule out hip pathology such as degenerative osteoarthritis. Lower extremity pulses should always be assessed to help differentiate vascular from neurogenic processes.

Older patients with acute or persisting LBP or possible radicular symptoms warrant diagnostic evaluation. Standing plain radiographs to include flexion/extension views (to assess for scoliosis or spondylolisthesis) should be obtained. Plain radiographs of the pelvis can evaluate the hip joints for the presence of degenerative hip osteoarthritis. Magnetic resonance imaging (MRI) is the study of choice to evaluate the spinal canal for any actual stenosis (needed to truly make the diagnosis of LSS) and to identify the cause of any stenosis present. If an MRI is contraindicated, computed tomography (CT) can be used but can only reliably show the bony dimensions of the canal and not any soft tissue components contributing to canal stenosis (like ligaments, disc, or tumor). Adding myelography to the CT will allow for visualization of the degree of compression of the thecal sac, however. Electrodiagnosis (electromyography (EMG) and nerve conduction studies (NCS)) can be used as well. Although the true sensitivity and specificity of electrodiagnostic testing for LSS is not well-defined, it can identify axon loss associated with radiculopathy or the presence of a peripheral polyneuropathy or other neuromuscular disease. As the prevalence of these latter conditions increases with age, EMG and NCS can help with a more accurate neurological diagnosis than can be obtained by physical exam and imaging alone. Vascular evaluation such as an ankle-brachial index (ABI) may be indicated to evaluate for vascular disease.

Treatment options for LSS vary, and there are limited data on their utility. In general, recent guidelines recommend modified exercise (with or without physical therapy for guidance), manual therapy, and behavioral interventions (such as encouraging activity and addressing depression, anxiety, and isolation). Exercise typically involves modifications to allow for spinal flexion, such as using walking sticks, walking on a treadmill with a slight incline, using a recumbent bicycle, or aquatic therapy. Over the counter medications are generally not helpful, and gabapentinoids are similarly not recommended. There is some limited support for the use of tricyclic antidepressants (TCAs) and serotonin-norepinephrine reuptake inhibitors (SNRIs), although there are potential side effects with these. Despite being commonly used, there are actually good data that epidural steroid injections are *not* helpful, and they should not be part of the routine care of patients with LSS. The most important component of treatment of LSS is getting people moving, exercising, and engaging in home and social tasks on a routine basis. That may require working through barriers, fear, lack of access, depression, walking aids, and adaptations at home.

Beyond relatively uncommon urgent "red flag" situations, surgery is generally indicated for those with progressive neurological loss and marked functional decline due to pain. The most common operative technique is a posterior decompressive laminectomy. This technique focuses on enlarging the spinal canal to relieve pressure on the nerve roots. Although data are limited, surgery seems to be effective in the short term. Within 8–10 years, however, there is often progressive decline following surgery with little difference noted between surgical and nonsurgical groups. In the United States, there is a growing trend toward incorporating lumbar fusion into surgical care for those with LSS. Documentation of any added benefit of fusion is lacking, although there is clearly an increased risk of complications with fusion as opposed to an isolated laminectomy. The presence of a spondylolisthesis or scoliosis may alter surgical considerations. As with other spine procedures, Black patients tend to have higher complication rates with surgery for LSS and longer post-operative hospital stays than White patients. Again, there is no association between the severity of stenosis on imaging and surgical outcomes. Given the relatively favorable natural history noted above, clearly nonsurgical care is most appropriate for the majority of patients with LSS.

For the patient presented here, LSS is the dominant clinical concern. He has become more sedentary and gained weight, both of which are problematic. Clinical evaluation should be directed toward excluding vascular disease, hip pathology, or a peripheral polyneuropathy as described above. Assuming his neurological exam is normal, he needs to engage in an exercise program to address general fitness, range of motion, lower extremity and trunk strength, balance, and modified gait training to incorporate more lumbar flexion (such as the introduction of walking sticks, a recumbent bicycle, or a pool). Physical therapy to assist in these would be quite appropriate. Medications should largely be avoided, although a TCA or SNRI could be trialed for neuropathic pain/paresthesia if no medical contraindications are present. Depression, social and economic barriers to activity and rehabilitation, diet, and comorbidities should be addressed. Plain radiographs of his spine should be obtained, including standing flexion/extension views. If there is concern for vascular disease, hip pathology, or a peripheral polyneuropathy, ABIs, hip radiographs, or electrodiagnostic testing should be obtained, respectively. If he has no red flag concerns, is neurologically intact, and has not even begun an exercise program, there is no indication for surgery, no role for an epidural steroid injection, and no need for an MRI at this point.

KEY POINTS

1. There is an important difference between radiographic stenosis (anatomical narrowing) and the clinical syndrome of LSS.
2. The hallmark symptoms of the clinical syndrome of LSS is neurogenic claudication, meaning leg symptoms that increase with standing or walking and decrease with sitting or lumbar flexion.
3. The natural history of LSS is generally believed to be favorable, with most patients remaining stable or showing clinical improvement over several years.
4. Nonsurgical treatment should focus on exercise, education, adaptive gait training, addressing socioeconomic and psychological barriers toward exercise, and care for underlying fear, depression, anxiety, and isolation.

5. Surgery is largely reserved for those with progressive neurological loss or significant leg pain. The benefits of surgery decline with time.

Further reading

1. Comer C, Ammendolia C, Battié MC, et al. Consensus on a standardised treatment pathway algorithm for lumbar spinal stenosis: an international Delphi study. BMC Musculoskelet Disord. 2022 Jun 8;23(1):550. doi: 10.1186/s12891-022-05485-5. PMID: 35676677; PMCID: PMC9175311.
2. Friedly JL, Comstock BA, Turner JA, et al. A randomized trial of epidural glucocorticoid injections for spinal stenosis. N Engl J Med. 2014 Jul 3;371(1):11–21. doi: 10.1056/NEJMoa1313265. Erratum in: N Engl J Med. 2014 Jul 24;371(4):390. PMID: 24988555.
3. Genevay S, Atlas SJ. Lumbar spinal stenosis. Best Pract Res Clin Rheumatol. 2010 Apr;24(2):253–265. doi: 10.1016/j.berh.2009.11.001. PMID: 20227646; PMCID: PMC2841052.
4. Oster BA, Kikanloo SR, Levine NL, et al. Systematic review of outcomes following 10-year mark of Spine Patient Outcomes Research Trial (SPORT) for spinal stenosis. Spine (Phila Pa 1976). 2020 Jun 15;45(12):832–836. doi: 10.1097/BRS.0000000000003323. PMID: 31770345.
5. Wessberg P, Frennered K. Central lumbar spinal stenosis: natural history of non-surgical patients. Eur Spine J. 2017 Oct;26(10):2536–2542. doi: 10.1007/s00586-017-5075-x. Epub 2017 Apr 17. PMID: 28417234.

8 "They Told Me I Have a 'Spondy.'": A 52-Year-Old with Low Back Pain

Christopher J. Standaert,

Jaxon E. Standaert

A 52-year-old male presents after 3 weeks of axial low back pain (LBP). He has had several episodes of low back pain in the last 10 years, all self-limiting and none associated with leg pain or other radicular symptoms. He has never had any significant trauma to his spine. His medical history is otherwise notable only for hypertension. He works in customer service and is sedentary for most of his workday. He has no other concerning symptoms. Although he is about 50% better since the onset of his pain, he was concerned and went to an urgent care clinic last week. Radiographs of his lumbar spine were obtained. He was told he has a "spondy" with fractures in his spine. The formal report notes an isthmic spondylolisthesis, grade I, with bilateral fractures of the pars interarticularis. This has him even more concerned, and he has been very cautious with his activity. He wants to know what happened to his spine and what he should do.

What do you do now?

sthmic spondylolisthesis is a relatively common finding on radiographic studies. It is not associated with or typically a cause of LBP in adults, however, and patients with axial LBP and radiographs showing spondylolysis or an isthmic spondylolisthesis should generally be treated the same as those who do not have similar findings.

Spondylolisthesis is defined as the anterior displacement of one vertebral body over the subjacent vertebral body. In origin, the prefix "spondylo" means "vertebra." The suffix "lysis" means a break or disruption, and "listhesis" means "slip." The word "spondylolisthesis" thus can be loosely translated to patients as a "spine-slip."

Spondylolisthesis is typically viewed under the following classifications:

Type I—Dysplastic
Type II—Isthmic
Type III—Degenerative
Type IV—Traumatic
Type V—Pathological

From a clinical standpoint, isthmic and degenerative spondylolisthesis are the most commonly encountered of these (degenerative spondylolisthesis is addressed in chapter 9). Isthmic spondylolisthesis refers to conditions where a slip is associated with a defect or defects in the pars interarticularis of the neural arch of the vertebra. The pars fracture defect itself is termed "spondylolysis." Roughly 75% of those with bilateral pars fractures will develop an associated slip—an "isthmic spondylolisthesis" (see Figure 8.1). In this setting, there are fractures on both sides of the neural arch, so the vertebral body translates forward while the posterior portion of the arch does not, thus there is typically no effect on the spinal canal. Spinal canal stenosis is therefore uncommon in this population, which distinguishes this condition from degenerative spondylolisthesis, where spinal canal stenosis is common. Spondylolistheses are graded by the extent of the slip and measured as a percentage of the horizontal diameter of the subjacent vertebral body.

Grade 1: <25%
Grade 2: 26–50%
Grade 3: 51–75%
Grade 4: 76–100%
Grade 5 (spondyloptosis): >100%

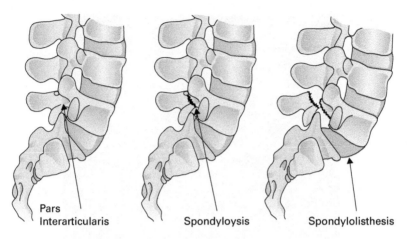

Pars
Interarticularis   Spondyloysis   Spondylolisthesis

FIGURE 8.1. Spondylolysis and isthmic spondylolisthesis.

The pars interarticularis (left) is a narrow bridge of bone found in the back portion of the vertebra. Spondylolysis (center) occurs when there is a fracture of the pars interarticularis. Spondylolisthesis (right) occurs when the vertebra shifts forward due to instability from the pars fracture.

Pars defects are noted on plain radiographs in about 6% of the adult population. This number appears to be slightly higher in studies using computed tomography (CT) scans. They occur about twice as often in men than in women and occur more commonly in Caucasians and those of Asian descent than in African Americans. Roughly 90% occur in the L5 vertebra, meaning that an associated slip, if present, occurs at L5/S1 (Figure 8.2). To better understand the natural history of spondylolysis and spondylolisthesis, investigators obtained plain radiographs on 500 first graders in Pennsylvania between the years 1955 and 1957 and subsequently published 45-year follow-up data on those with isthmic spondylolysis. The authors found pars fractures in 4.4% of the first graders (roughly age 6), all of whom were asymptomatic. That number increased to 6% by age 25. About 80% of those with bilateral pars fractures went on to develop a spondylolisthesis, while none of those with a unilateral pars fracture did. As the incidence of pars fractures in newborns or those who have never been ambulatory is zero, it is assumed that these fractures largely occur early in life, likely related to ambulation. This is true in the vast majority of those identified as having a pars fracture or isthmic spondylolisthesis on

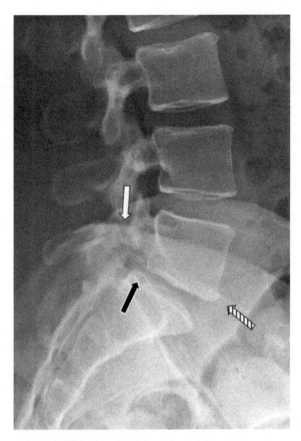

FIGURE 8.2. Plain lateral radiograph showing isthmic spondylolisthesis.

This radiograph shows a Grade 1 isthmic spondylolisthesis at L5/S1 (black arrow) with disc height loss. Pars defects (white arrow) and anterior osteophytes (striped arrow) are present at L5.

radiographs, which can be challenging to explain to patients seeing a report of their radiographs.

There has been debate as to whether or not pars fractures or an associated spondylolisthesis are causes of back pain in adults. From multiple studies, it seems clear that they are not generally a cause of axial LBP, and those with these radiographic findings have rates of LBP that are identical to comparative populations without spondylolysis or isthmic spondylolisthesis. Additionally, the prevalence of isthmic spondylolysis or isthmic spondylolisthesis does not seem to change after age 20. New isthmic fractures not related to other spine pathology or trauma are thus rare, if they even occur, in the adult population. It is important to explain to patients that an existing isthmic spondylolisthesis on radiographs most likely occurred early in their childhood and is also most likely unrelated to any axial LBP that they are experiencing.

Many patients and clinicians have concern regarding the potential for progression of the slip in those with isthmic spondylolisthesis. For the most part, the greatest degree of slip occurs during adolescence. Some adults will have slip progression and many will have degeneration of the disc at the level of the slip. However, slip progression of greater than 10 mm occurs in less than 5% of adults with isthmic spondylolisthesis (for reference, a typical adult vertebral body has an antero-posterior diameter of about 40 mm, so 10 mm represents an additional 25% slip). In general, most adults with an asymptomatic isthmic spondylolisthesis can be assured that there is a very low risk that their slip will progress to any significant degree.

The patient presented here has axial LBP without radiation or any neurologic concerns. Given the existing data, his isthmic spondylolisthesis likely began in early childhood, without any symptoms, and is unrelated to his chronic, recurrent LBP. He is at low risk for slip progression or future significant problems related to his isthmic spondylolisthesis. Evaluation should be directed toward excluding neurologic compromise, particularly L5 nerve root involvement, assessing for other unrelated processes which may be associated with his pain, and assessing his degree of functional impairment and potential barriers to improvement so treatment can be initiated.

Physical examination should include palpation of the spine, assessment for coexistent scoliosis or similar issues, and neurologic examination. As with all patients with LBP, a neurologic examination of his lower extremities including motor, sensory, and reflex function is required. In this case, particular attention should be paid to muscles typically innervated by the L5 nerve root, including ankle dorsiflexion (tibialis anterior) and great toe extension (extensor hallucis longus).

Several diagnostic studies could be considered in patients with isthmic spondylolisthesis. In this case, his spondylolisthesis was identified by plain radiographs. If there are concerns for instability, standing flexion/

extension radiographs can also be obtained. Although oblique lumbar radiographs are more sensitive in identifying pars lesions than antero-posterior and lateral views, their value is questionable, as identification of a pars fracture without a spondylolisthesis does not typically change clinical management given the data cited above. Magnetic resonance imaging (MRI) is generally not required or indicated in the evaluation of axial LBP. In the setting of isthmic spondylolisthesis, the typical indication for MRI would be the presence of leg pain suggesting nerve root involvement, concern for an underlying radiculopathy with weakness or numbness, or concern for other significant pathology (tumor, infection, etc.). As isthmic spondylolisthesis does not typically cause spinal canal stenosis, the relevant pathology is most often narrowing of the neural foramen at the level of the spondylolisthesis. CT can occasionally be helpful in assessing or clarifying the presence of a pars defect or other bone pathology. If a patient has radiating leg pain or neurologic concerns, electrodiagnostic testing can be considered to evaluate for the presence of a lumbar radiculopathy or other lower motor neuron processes. In the current case, in which the patient has only axial LBP with no other concerning symptoms or neurologic loss, there is no indication for any further imaging or diagnostic evaluation.

Treatment for this patient should be focused on getting him active. Given the potential deleterious effects of fear avoidance or "medicalization" of his LBP, this patient needs reassurance of the benign and preexisting nature of his isthmic spondylolisthesis. He needs to recognize that roughly 1 in 20 males his age have the same thing, and that they are all are at no more risk than anyone else for LBP.

His treatment should follow the same approach as for other individuals with chronic recurrent LBP (see chapter 2). In the acute setting, activity within tolerance should be encouraged. Structured exercise can be beneficial, whatever form that may take. In general, active exercise programs are beneficial in patients with chronic recurrent LBP, and there is no single exercise program that has been shown to be uniquely effective. The benefits of exercise appear to extend beyond simply the physiologic response to specific tasks, and exercise is associated with a lower frequency and severity of recurrences of LBP. There is no evidence available on the role of medications, spinal manipulation, corticosteroid injections, bracing, traction, or transcutaneous electrical stimulation (TENS) in the treatment of isthmic spondylolisthesis. The presence of an isthmic spondylolistheses presents no additional indications for any of these modalities.

The situation changes clinically if a patient with isthmic spondylolisthesis is experiencing radiating leg pain/sciatica, weakness, or numbness. An isthmic spondylolisthesis can be associated with narrowing of the adjacent neural foramen, and there can be compromise of the exiting nerve root or roots at that level. As the vast majority of isthmic spondylolistheses occur at L5/S1, pain and neurologic issues typically arise from compromise of the L5 root in the neural foramen. Pain and numbness are usually noted in the lateral calf and dorsum of the foot, and weakness of ankle dorsiflexion and great toe extension (along with other muscles with L5 innervation) may occur.

There is significant uncertainty about the role of surgery in treating isthmic spondylolisthesis. Surgical indications include progressive neurologic loss and intractable pain, particularly radicular pain. Although studies generally show significant clinical improvement for patients undergoing lumbar fusion, there are insufficient data to assess the relative benefits of differing surgical approaches in treating isthmic spondylolisthesis. Surgery should primarily be considered in those with significant, intractable radicular pain or neurologic loss that correlates with the level of their spondylolisthesis and other diagnostic findings.

There are data on the relative prevalence of isthmic spondylolisthesis in variety of populations, including Caucasians, African Americans, Inuit and related populations, and those in a number of Asian countries. In general, the prevalence of spondylolysis is similar in Caucasian and Asian populations, lower in African American populations (2.3% for males, 1.1% for females), and markedly higher (20–60%) in Inuit populations. The prevalence in males is roughly twice that in females across populations. There are limited data on specific treatment outcomes in all populations. High level data on differential outcomes or rates of intervention by demographic variables are lacking. Although spondylolysis is almost entirely an asymptomatic radiographic finding in adults, more data or research on the differential responses to treatment among differing ethnicities or between males and females would be helpful.

1. Isthmic spondylolysis with or without spondylolisthesis is seen on plain radiographs of the lumbar spine in about 6% of people.
2. The radiographic findings of isthmic spondylolisthesis are generally not associated with or a cause of LBP in adults.
3. The fractures related to isthmic spondylolisthesis occur primarily in childhood without symptoms.
4. Isthmic spondylolisthesis occurs twice as often in men compared to women.
5. The vast majority of isthmic spondylolistheses occur at L5/S1.

Further reading

1. Andrade NS, Ashton CM, Wray NP, Brown C, Bartanusz V. Systematic review of observational studies reveals no association between low back pain and lumbar spondylolysis with or without isthmic spondylolisthesis. Eur Spine J. 2015 Jun;24(6):1289–1295. doi: 10.1007/s00586-015-3910-5. Epub 2015 Apr 2. PMID: 25833204.
2. Beutler WJ, Fredrickson BE, Murtland A, Sweeney CA, Grant WD, Baker D. The natural history of spondylolysis and spondylolisthesis: 45-year follow-up evaluation. Spine (Phila Pa 1976). 2003 May 15;28(10):1027–1035; discussion 1035. doi: 10.1097/01.BRS.0000061992.98108.A0. PMID: 12768144.
3. Fredrickson BE, Baker D, McHolick WJ, Yuan HA, Lubicky JP. The natural history of spondylolysis and spondylolisthesis. J Bone Joint Surg Am. 1984 Jun;66(5):699–707. PMID: 6373773.
4. Kreiner DS, Baisden J, Mazanec DJ, et al. Guideline summary review: an evidence-based clinical guideline for the diagnosis and treatment of adult isthmic spondylolisthesis. Spine J. 2016 Dec;16(12):1478–1485. doi: 10.1016/j.spinee.2016.08.034. Epub 2016 Sep 1. PMID: 27592807.
5. Roche MB, Rowe GG. The incidence of separate neural arch and coincident bone variations; a survey of 4,200 skeletons. Anat Rec. 1951 Feb;109(2):233–252. doi: 10.1002/ar.1091090207. PMID: 14811059.

9 A "Clunk" in the Night: A 51-Year-Old Female with Back Pain

Joseph P. Shivers,

Christopher J. Standaert

A patient whom you have seen for several years comes in for evaluation of intermittent low back pain. She is 51, relatively thin with a BMI of 21, and is a small animal veterinarian in town. She likes to walk and practices yoga off and on. She has had some degree of back pain since her mid-40s, predominantly in her lower lumbar spine. She has found work progressively more challenging with all of the bending and reaching involved in caring for animals. Most recently, she has noticed an almost audible "clunk" sensation in her back when she rolls over at night. She does not have significant leg pain but notes rare paresthesias into her legs. She is not eager to take medication. She feels as though she is relatively healthy and wants to keep working for many years. She is concerned by the sensation she experiences at night and the difficulty with working. Stretching and yoga do not really seem to help.

What do you do now?

This patient is a woman in her early 50s with several years of worsening axial back pain that is exacerbated by bending and reaching. She also has intermittent paresthesias of the bilateral lower extremities and recently has experienced a "clunk" sensation with turning over in bed. There are no red-flag symptoms that would warrant advanced imaging or surgical consultation, or yellow-flag symptoms that would merit further psychosocial exploration. This history is not diagnostic in itself. However, it does suggest a degenerative spondylolisthesis.

Spondylolisthesis, from the Greek spondylo (spine) + olisthesis (slip), is an anatomical term that describes a misalignment of two vertebrae in the sagittal plane. Normally, when the lumbar spine is viewed laterally, there is a gentle lordotic curve that can be traced along the posterior aspect of each vertebral body. However, in a spondylolisthesis, one vertebra has "slipped" forward relative to the vertebra below, so that between these two vertebrae, the smooth imaginary line is sharply interrupted (see Figure 9.1A).

Spondylolistheses can be categorized by their anatomy and etiology. In a degenerative spondylolisthesis, the underlying problem seems to be laxity in the facet joints, which would normally help to restrict intervertebral motion in the sagittal plane. At a given intervertebral level, the right and left facet joints (zygapophysial joints) are part of the posterior elements of the spine. They are capsular joints formed between the inferior articular processes of the vertebra above and the superior articular processes of the vertebra below. When the facet joints are too lax, the vertebra above can gradually shift forward relative to the vertebra below. Over time, the facet joints show radiological evidence of wear and tear, which can be referred to as arthritis, arthrosis, hypertrophy, or arthropathy. The intervertebral disc can be degenerative at this level as well, although disc changes seem most likely to be secondary.

Over time, the progression of degenerative spondylolisthesis tends to slow down and stop, in association with arthritic changes, such as disc-height loss, bone spurring (osteophytosis), and ossification of the posterior longitudinal ligament. However, if the spondylolisthesis progresses enough, it can contribute to a focal narrowing of the spinal canal (i.e. lumbar spinal stenosis).

Degenerative spondylolisthesis is characterized by a chronic, gradual, and imperceptible shift of one vertebra relative to the one below it. However,

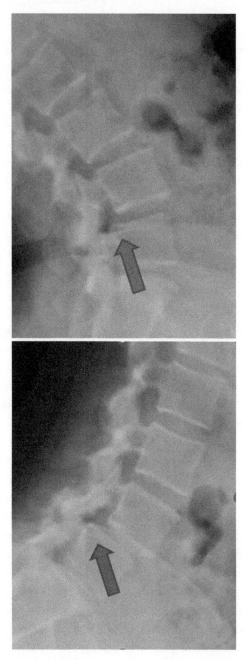

FIGURES 9.1A AND 9.1B. Standing flexion/extension X-rays showing a degenerative spondylolisthesis. The film on the left is in extension (A) and shows a small listhesis ("slip") at L4/L5 (arrow). The film on the right is in flexion (B) and shows mild increase in the listhesis ("slip"), consistent with mild instability. Note that the vertebrae above maintain their alignment.

the patient's lax joints can also allow small sudden shifts back and forth. For example, in lumbar flexion, the vertebra above can slide further forward; whereas with lumbar extension, it would slide back again (see Figures 9.1A and B). A positional shift of this sort is sometimes called a dynamic listhesis or dynamic instability. Dynamic instability can sometimes be perceived by the patient as a sense of shifting or clunking in the back itself. Patients might also describe the intermittent sensation of lower extremity numbness, tingling, or pain, attributable to positional nerve-root irritation. The most common symptom of degenerative spondylolisthesis, with or without a dynamic component, is simply chronic axial low back pain (LBP).

Degenerative spondylolisthesis is more common in women than men, more common in African Americans than Caucasians, and more common after age 50 than before. It also seems to be more common in people who are diffusely hypermobile, and there may be increased risk in occupations that involve a lot of bending. It occurs most often at the L4/L5 level, and less often at L3/L4, L5/S1, or elsewhere. Degenerative spondylolisthesis is not always symptomatic. However, in a patient with LBP who is found to have degenerative spondylolisthesis, the slippage and associated degenerative changes probably *are* relevant to the understanding and management of their spine. This is in contrast to isthmic spondylolisthesis, which in skeletally mature adults is almost never a cause of back pain (see chapter 8).

In teaching patients about the management options for degenerative spondylolisthesis, we often use the following analogy. Imagine that the spine is a column of bricks, built to hold up the deck of a house. A degenerative spondylolisthesis is like the bricks slipping forward at one place in the tower. To stabilize the column of bricks, there are three general approaches. One way is to tightly wrap the tower in sheet metal. The second way is to replace the mortar in between the bricks. The third way is to anchor the top of the column with guy-wires.

The three strategies in the analogy correspond to three categories of real-world management options. Wrapping the column in sheet metal is like wearing a lumbar brace. A lumbar brace, by providing external support, can increase comfort during activities that are known to provoke symptoms (e.g. occupational lifting, yard work, playing with small children). However, if the brace is worn for several hours or more at a time, then the stabilizing trunk muscles can get weaker, which would be counterproductive.

Replacing the mortar is analogous to spinal fusion surgery. Surgery seems intuitive at the conceptual level: if the problem is that the intervertebral joints are too loose, then why not fuse the vertebrae together? The problems are that spine surgeries come with some degree of risk, and they often do not improve axial back pain. Also, in the setting of this underlying degenerative process, a fusion at one level does not protect the adjacent vertebral levels from degeneration. Surgery tends to be warranted in two general cases. The first case for surgery is when, despite appropriate physical therapy, the degenerative spondylolisthesis is causing severe and worsening symptomatic lumbar radiculopathy or lumbar spinal stenosis (i.e. buttock or leg pain more so than back pain, worse with standing and walking, better with forward flexion, quickly relieved after sitting down—see chapter 7). The second general case where surgery may be warranted is if there is significant LBP with severe dynamic instability. Definitions vary, but many would say that this entails >5mm of shift between flexion and extension on standing X-rays. Otherwise, nonsurgical management tends to be best.

Returning once more to the analogy of the brick column, adding tension with guy-wires is like training and strengthening the muscles that stabilize the trunk. This approach should be the mainstay of treatment for degenerative spondylolisthesis. The concept tends to be readily comprehensible by patients. There is a problem with some of the stabilizing structures (the facet joints, maybe the disc), so the solution is to improve the function of other stabilizing structures (muscles). To the best of our knowledge, which forms of exercise are best for people with degenerative spondylolisthesis has not been definitively determined by clinical trials. However, in our clinical experience, people seem to do better with exercise programs that emphasize stability and precise control of movement (e.g. isometric PT exercises, Pilates) as opposed to programs directed toward increasing flexibility (e.g. stretching-based PT exercises, many varieties of yoga).

We mentioned above that patients with degenerative spondylolisthesis are often more mobile than the general population. It seems that these patients are also disproportionately likely to already be doing things like stretching and yoga, as is the patient in this case. These activities further improve the patient's excellent flexibility but do relatively little to address their stability. This pattern is illustrative of two larger principles that we sometimes teach patients: "People don't get hurt because of what they are good at, they get hurt because of what they are bad at" and "Left to their own devices, people tend to do what they are good at." The challenge for the patient becomes how to redirect some of their energies toward shoring up their weaknesses. They can do this by finding new activities that they inherently enjoy ("It turns out I really like Pilates"), modifying their old activities ("My back feels so much better since I replaced the deep stretches in my morning flow routine with more static poses"), or by consciously linking therapeutic exercise to the activity they do prefer ("My PT exercises are boring, but if I do them consistently two to three times a week, then I'm able to do yoga on the other days without much pain").

For people seeking relief of axial back pain despite the biomechanical tactics above and despite reasonable pharmacology (e.g. nonsteroidal anti-inflammatory drugs (NSAIDs)), some interventional procedures are available. The first is radiofrequency ablation (RFA) of the medial branches that carry pain signals from the affected facet joints. The advantage of RFA is that pain is relieved until the medial branch regrows—up to 1 year in many cases. The chief downside is that the medial branch also innervates the multifidus muscle, part of the stabilizing musculature in the back—which seems counterproductive in a disease state where the key management principle is to strengthen the stabilizing musculature. The other broad category of procedure is intra-articular injection of corticosteroid into the arthritic facet joints themselves. Intra-articular injections have the advantage of not compromising the stabilizing musculature, but they do involve some degree of systemic steroid exposure, not to mention potential chondrotoxic effects within the joint.

Other points of note are that weight loss intuitively makes sense from a biomechanical perspective in a patient who is obese, and work-duty modification makes sense if a person's job exacerbates their symptoms.

Let's return to the case of this woman for whom a degenerative spondylolisthesis seems likely based on the history. On physical exam she can touch her fingertips to the ground while keeping her knees extended. In palpating the lumbar spine, there is no palpable "step-off." Such a step-off would be relatively specific but not sensitive for focal alignment issues in the sagittal plane.

The next step is to obtain standing X-rays of the lumbar spine in four views: anterior-posterior in neutral stance, lateral in neutral stance, lateral in lumbar flexion, and lateral in lumbar extension. The X-rays confirm the diagnosis of degenerative spondylolisthesis, L4 on L5. In the neutral lateral view, comparing the posterior aspects of the L4 and L5 vertebrae, L4 is 3 millimeters more anterior. In the extension view, this difference remains at 3 mm, whereas in flexion, the difference is 6 mm. Thus, she has a static spondylolisthesis of 3 mm and an additional dynamic slippage of 3 mm. For context, the margin of error on plain radiographs is 2 mm. The patient's radiographs are also notable for blurriness and irregularity of the facet joints at L4/L5, though the facet joint lines are crisp at L3/L4. Disc heights are generally well maintained, though a bit of disc height seems to have been lost at L4/L5 and L5/S1 (see Figure 9.1B).

For this patient we would recommend a physical therapy regimen that begins with static core stabilization and closed kinetic-chain trunk exercises, with progression to more dynamic exercises targeted to her relatively physical job. Depending on her progress with physical therapy and the status of her lower extremity symptoms, we might support her in seeking a schedule modification so that she has more help from colleagues with managing animals of a certain weight. We would suggest that she try wearing a brace during periods of dynamic exertion (e.g. periods of an hour or two at a time when she'll be lifting animals at work). If she were to develop symptomatic lumbar stenosis and/or lumbar radiculopathy, we would obtain repeat standing X-rays of the lumbar spine including flexion/extension views as well as a lumbar MRI, and we would consider a surgical referral. In this patient, who is not interested in pharmacologic management, we would not prescribe any medications. We would be cautiously optimistic for a good long-term outcome with this strategy, but we would also make sure that she understands the signs and symptoms of neurologic compromise that should prompt her to contact us for timely reevaluation.

KEY POINTS

1. Degenerative spondylolisthesis is characterized by an anterior slip of one vertebra relative to the vertebra below, most commonly at L4/L5, in the setting of wear and tear ("degenerative") changes of the facet joints. Risk factors

include age greater than 50, female sex, African American race, and generalized above average joint flexibility.

2. The most common presenting symptom associated with degenerative spondylolisthesis is LBP, although patients may also experience symptomatic spinal stenosis, radicular lower extremity symptoms, and/or perceptible instability (e.g. the "clunk" in this case description).

3. Radiologic evaluation of a patient with possible degenerative spondylolisthesis should include standing X-rays of the standing patient's lumbar spine, including an anterior-posterior view and three lateral views: neutral stance, lumbar forward flexion, and lumbar extension.

4. The core of nonoperative management is to improve the strength, endurance, and coordination of the stabilizing muscles of the trunk and lumbopelvic junction. Judicious use of a lumbar brace, for an hour or so at a time, may also be helpful.

5. Operative indications include progressive lower extremity neurologic changes, despite an appropriate trial of conservative management, and severe low back pain accompanied by severe dynamic instability.

Further reading

1. Kalichman L, Hunter DJ. Diagnosis and conservative management of degenerative lumbar spondylolisthesis. Eur Spine J. 2008;17:327–335. doi: 10.1007/s00586-007-0543-3.

2. Jacobsen S, Sonne-Holm S, Rovsing H, Monrad H, Gebuhr P. Degenerative lumbar spondylolisthesis: an epidemiological perspective: the Copenhagen Osteoarthritis Study. Spine (Phila Pa 1976). 2007;32(1):120–125. doi: 10.1097/01.brs.0000250979.12398.96.

3. Matsunaga S, Sakou T, Morizono Y, Masuda A, Demirtas AM. Natural history of degenerative spondylolisthesis: pathogenesis and natural course of the slippage. Spine (Phila Pa 1976). 1990;15(11):1204–1210. doi: 10.1097/00007632-199011010-00021.

4. Mannion AF, Pittet V, Steiger F, Vader J-P, Becker H-J, Porchet F. The Zurich Appropriateness of Spine Surgery (ZASS) Group. Development of appropriateness criteria for the surgical treatment of lumbar degenerative spondylolisthesis (LDS). Eur Spine J. 2014;23:1903–1917. doi: 10.1007/s00586-014-3284-0.

10 "My Back Aches, and I Can't Stand Long Enough to Make Dinner.": Chronic Low Back Pain at 73

Michelle Eventov, Christopher J. Standaert

A 73-year-old female, long-established with your practice, presents with diffuse back pain that has become more limiting over a few years. She describes pain throughout her back that increases with standing. She can only stand still a few minutes before pain and fatigue force her to sit. She cannot stand long enough to cook a full meal. She is more comfortable walking but fatigues with that as well. She can walk better when leaning on a shopping cart. There was no injury or trauma. She has no leg pain or neurologic complaints. She feels like she stoops forward more than she used to and that her clothes don't fit the same. She attends a Silver Sneakers exercise class twice per week. She has osteopenia, hypertension, and hypothyroidism, all of which are stable. On examination you note a scoliosis that seems more prominent than you recall. There is no focal tenderness in her back. She is underweight but relatively healthy-appearing for age with a normal neurologic examination.

What do you do now?

The differential diagnosis of low back pain (LBP) in a 73-year-old is broad, but this patient is describing progressive scoliosis. Degenerative scoliosis develops during adulthood, arising from a range of degenerative phenomena in the lumbar spine. It is commonly associated with LBP with or without radicular symptoms. Given her age and history of osteopenia, this patient will require a thorough evaluation to exclude concerning pathology such as a compression fracture or neoplasm. Assuming there are no acute concerns, it is important to understand the nature of and treatment for adult degenerative scoliosis.

Scoliosis is defined by a Cobb angle >10°. This angle measures the spine's lateral curvature in the coronal plane, as seen in an antero-posterior (A/P) standing radiograph (Figure 10.1). Although the definition is in one plane, scoliosis is a three-dimensional process, affecting global alignment. Adult scoliosis is categorized as idiopathic or degenerative. Idiopathic adult scoliosis is the continuation of an adolescent idiopathic scoliosis and is not typically associated with LBP. Degenerative scoliosis is acquired in adulthood and is a result of progressive asymmetric degenerative change. Idiopathic lumbar scoliotic curves are typically accompanied by compensatory thoracic curves, resulting in relative balance of the spine. In comparison, degenerative lumbar scoliosis generally occurs without a compensatory curve and is thus more prone to relative "imbalance."

Degenerative scoliosis affects close to half of the older adult population. It presents around age 70, and its prevalence is linearly correlated with age between 40 and 90. There is no difference in prevalence between males and females, however females have more rapid progression after menopause due to accelerated loss of bone density. Caucasians have a higher rate of degenerative scoliosis than any other ethnic group. In one study, African Americans were shown to have milder cases compared to other races. LBP is present in 60% or more of individuals with degenerative scoliosis. Spinal stenosis, radicular pain, pain with standing or walking, postural changes, and height loss can also occur. Rarely, patients may present with dyspnea due to thoracic involvement causing a restrictive lung pattern.

When gathering a history, one should ask about risk factors for degenerative scoliosis. These include prior spine surgeries, osteoporosis, spinal cord injury, certain polyneuropathies, cerebral palsy, and diseases affecting

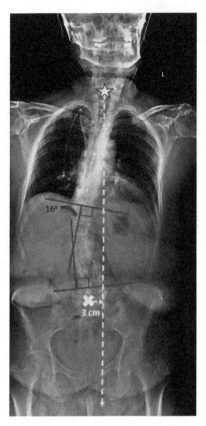

FIGURE 10.1. Antero-posterior (A/P) full-length radiograph. The solid lines measure a Cobb angle of 16° between the inferior endplate of T10 to the inferior endplate of L4. The dashed lines measure the coronal balance. The vertical dashed line drops down from the middle of the C7 vertebral body (star). This should pass through the middle of S1 (X). In this case, the vertical line passes to the left of midline. This patient has a 3 cm coronal imbalance to the left.

collagen. Conditions that may contribute to leg length discrepancies, such as prior lower limb surgery, amputation, or hip dysplasia, can also increase risk.

The differential diagnosis of LBP is broad but includes muscle strain, facet arthropathy, osteoporotic vertebral fracture, and disc herniation. A practitioner should always look for red flags such as saddle anesthesia, new weakness, and bowel or bladder dysfunction, as these may be signs of acute spinal cord or cauda equina compression.

On physical examination for those with scoliosis, assess for lateral asymmetries of the back, shoulders, hips, and arm lengths. You should also inspect from the side to appreciate the degree of kyphosis or lordosis. Ask the patient to perform an Adam's forward bend test where they bend at the waist while maintaining straight legs. Lateral asymmetries in thoracic or lumbar prominences when viewed from behind the patient are a sign of scoliosis. Inspection is followed by palpation of the spine and hips. Tenderness over bony prominences, especially in older adults, may indicate an underlying fracture. The neurologic exam (including strength, sensation, reflexes, and gait analysis) should be completed in order to rule out myelopathy or radiculopathy.

If the physical exam shows any signs of scoliosis, spine radiographs (standing A/P and lateral views) should be evaluated. These are ordered as scoliosis or "full cassette" films and run from the base of the skull to the pelvis. They must be obtained with the patient standing without external support. Scoliosis is confirmed by measuring a Cobb angle of >10° on the A/P image (see Figure 10.1). From the lateral radiograph, sagittal imbalance parameters can also be determined. A positive sagittal imbalance effectively translates to the head and neck being positioned anteriorly to the pelvis, resulting in significant difficulty maintaining an upright posture (see Figure 10.2). Sagittal spinopelvic alignment is a primary determinant of health-related quality of life measures. Even though Cobb angle defines scoliosis, it is not strongly correlated with disability. Rarely, magnetic resonance imaging is done for initial evaluation, usually when one has neurologic findings concerning for spinal cord compression or nerve impingement.

Gravity and time are the enemies of degenerative scoliosis. The imbalance of gravitational forces and the length of time these forces are applied contribute to curve progression. Without treatment, the rate of curve progression averages up to 1–2° per year. Factors associated with more rapid progression include Cobb angle >30°, the presence of a lumbar curve or lateral listhesis >6 mm, history of decompressive laminectomy or spinal fusion, and postmenopausal state in women. Age is not correlated with progression, despite being strongly correlated with the initial diagnosis.

The fundamental principles of managing scoliosis are maintaining postural endurance, spinal flexibility, appropriate weight, and healthy bone density. Poor physical condition or motor function will impair someone's

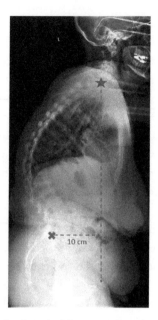

FIGURE 10.2. Lateral (sagittal) radiograph of the same patient shown in Figure 10.1 demonstrating sagittal imbalance. The vertical dashed line drops down from the middle of the C7 vertebral body (star). This should pass through the posterior aspect of S1 (X). In this case, the vertical line passes anteriorly to this point. This patient has a 10 cm positive sagittal imbalance with associated lumbar hyperlordosis and thoracic hyperkyphosis.

ability to "fight gravity," and less flexibility translates to a lower capacity to achieve spinal balance. The vast majority of older adults with degenerative scoliosis are managed nonoperatively with surgery reserved for those with severe functional impairment. Although nonsteroidal anti-inflammatory drugs (NSAIDs) and non-opioid analgesics may provide some pain relief, they have little utility in treatment. Gabapentinoids and opiates are also not recommended. Instead, practitioners should focus on movement and function. Below are many examples of therapies and techniques that target just that. The approach to scoliosis care should include a combination of these treatments that work synergistically to improve function.

Physical therapy is used to strengthen musculature for postural support and improve gait mechanics. Gait disturbances can create asymmetric forces that may enhance curve progression. The Schroth technique, developed in Germany in the 1800s, focuses on de-rotation, elongation, and stabilization of the spine in all three dimensions by increasing muscular symmetry, teaching rotational angular breathing (breathing into the concave side of the curve), and teaching postural awareness. Although developed for children, these approaches seem to translate to adults. The intent is to improve function rather than reverse curvature. Aquatic therapy is another variation that can mitigate the force of gravity. This allows patients to perform aerobic training and use a wide range of musculature while minimizing impact on the spine.

Pilates and modified yoga have also been shown to have benefit. There is some evidence demonstrating improvement in pain with chiropractic care. There is no evidence for improvement in Cobb angle or reversal of the scoliosis with spinal manipulation, however. Other alternative modalities such as massage and acupuncture can be tried on an individualized basis. However, as with chiropractic care, any benefit may be very short-term (hours to days), and the evidence supporting their utility is limited.

Bracing can be helpful in select scenarios. It may be beneficial if someone needs support to complete a task (e.g. preparing a meal). However, bracing should not be overutilized, as extensive use may lead to deconditioning that will increase instability and curve progression.

As with other conditions, walkers and canes are useful for providing stability. They can reduce pain, improve mobility, and decrease falls. In patients with limited functional capacity, rollator walkers can also provide a seat when needed. Pacing is a strategy that can be useful to many patients. The goal is to even out activity peaks and troughs in order to reduce fear avoidance (when one is fearful that an activity may cause pain) and overexertion (which often leads to "bad days" and reduced mobility). First, individuals must determine the length of time they can tolerate in a given posture or with a given activity. Daily tasks should be separated into segments within this level of tolerance. Thus, time is guiding activity duration rather than symptoms. Simple home modifications can also be helpful. For example, for those who cannot tolerate standing for meal preparation, keep a stool in the kitchen. As with other conditions that affect balance, remove any tripping hazards, such as loose rugs, in order to reduce falls.

Body weight is an important component of scoliosis care, as the force of gravity depends on mass. In those with an elevated body mass index (BMI), there is more force on the spine and thus the potential for further curve progression and functional decline. However, a low BMI can be a sign of low bone density, which poses a risk for fracture, as well as inadequate nutrition and protein stores with sarcopenia and loss of lean muscle mass. Bone mineral density should be assessed, and those with low density should be referred for treatment.

There is no specific curve severity or curve progression rate that deems someone a surgical candidate. Pain, functional impairment, bone density, and comorbidities are factors contributing to surgical decision-making. The goals of surgery are to decompress lumbar nerve roots, fuse unstable segments, and reestablish balance. Currently, there are no clear guidelines on which surgical procedure yields the best results. Complications of surgery include neurological injury, loss of spinal balance, degeneration of adjacent spinal segments, surgical site infections, and reoperation. In adults over age 66, complication rates for scoliosis surgery are 24% within 90 days with 13% requiring readmission within 30 days, and 12% requiring reoperation within 5 years. Surgical mortality rate is approximately 1%.

As with its treatment, the focus of monitoring scoliosis should be placed on function. Thus, there is little utility in repeating radiographs routinely. Instead, a clinician can utilize validated subjective measures, such as the Oswestry Disability Index or a variety of Patient Reported Outcomes Measurement Information System (PROMIS) scales that are publicly available and well validated. The Scoliosis Research Society has also developed a 22-point questionnaire focusing on pain, function, mood, relationships, self-image, and medication use.

Back to our case: this patient needs full-length standing scoliosis radiographs with measurements of Cobb angle as well as coronal and sagittal balance. Unless recently performed, she also should have a bone density scan with referral for treatment if needed. She should continue with regular exercise but should be referred to physical therapy for education about her curve, approaches to exercise, balance, and use of adaptive devices for gait. She should also be referred to occupational therapy for assistance with activities of daily living and for advice on safe and effective function in her home. If available and otherwise appropriate for her, aquatic exercise and/or aquatic physical therapy may be helpful. She can be provided with a soft lumbar brace to be used sparingly for specific tasks, such as cooking. She should also keep a stool in her kitchen and utilize pacing to complete household tasks. With her sagittal imbalance, a rollator walker may be helpful as her pain is improved with support while leaning forward. This will also assist with pacing, as it will provide a seat for her timed breaks. Over the counter analgesics and topical agents like superficial heat can be used for pain, but opiates, gabapentinoids, and other medications that impair cognition or safety should be avoided. Exercise, functional strategies, adaptive aids, dietary optimization, and education are the cornerstones of care.

KEY POINTS

1. Degenerative scoliosis is defined by a Cobb angle >10°. Despite this definition involving a coronal measurement, the presence of sagittal imbalance has a greater effect on disability.
2. Gravity and time are the enemies of scoliosis.
3. Treatment should be focused on function: gait mechanics, home setup, and activity modification are essential.
4. Weight is an important aspect of management. High BMI will increase the asymmetric force that gravity places on the spine, leading to progression of disease. Low BMI may be an indicator of low bone density, which can increase the risk of fracture.

Further reading

1. Ailon T, Smith J, Shaffrey C, et al. Degenerative spinal deformity. Neurosurgery. 2015;77:S75–S91.
2. Everett C, Patel R. A systematic literature review of nonsurgical treatment in adult scoliosis. Spine. 2007;32(Supplement):S130–S134.
3. Glassman S, Bridwell K, Dimar J, Horton W, Berven S, Schwab F. The impact of positive sagittal balance in adult spinal deformity. Spine. 2005;30(18):2024–2029.
4. Kotwal S, Pumberger M, Hughes A, Girardi F. Degenerative scoliosis: a review. HSS Journal. 2011;7(3):257–264.
5. Tribus C. Degenerative lumbar scoliosis: evaluation and management. J Am Acad Orthop Surg. 2003;11(3):174–183.

11 "I Shouldn't Have Moved That Flowerpot.": Acute Back Pain in a 78-Year-Old Woman

James E. Eubanks, Jr., Christopher J. Standaert

An uncomfortable 78-year-old female presents for evaluation of acute low back pain (LBP). The pain started five days ago, shortly after moving a large flowerpot on her patio. The pain is in her low back to sacral area. She is comfortable sitting or sleeping curled up on her side. Standing up straight is painful, and lifting anything causes more pain. She can get herself dressed and manage simple home tasks, but it hurts more to vacuum or make her bed. Her significant other has been doing all the home tasks since her pain started. She has a history of a hysterectomy in her 40s and coronary artery disease that is well managed. She never smoked but did have significant alcohol intake through her early 30s. She has been sober for decades. She walks around her block most days for exercise. Her last mammogram

and colonoscopy were unremarkable and performed
five years ago. A bone density study three years
ago showed osteopenia, and she is taking a calcium
supplement.

What do you do now?

A ny older adult presenting with acute, severe LBP warrants an urgent and thorough evaluation. Unlike with younger, low-risk individuals, these patients should be assumed to have significant pathology, such as a fracture or tumor, until proven otherwise. This case warrants urgent evaluation and imaging.

This patient's history is concerning for a vertebral compression fracture (VCF). VCFs involve a loss of vertebral body height due to excessive axial or compressive load and are most often secondary to weakening of the vertebral body due to osteoporosis. They may be associated with trauma, metastasis, or osteomyelitis, and identifying the cause and acuity of VCFs is necessary to ensure appropriate treatment. VCFs affect over 700,000 Americans each year and may negatively impact quality of life due to their association with subsequent fragility fractures and debility. With approximately 25% of postmenopausal females estimated to have at least one VCF, they are the most common of all osteoporotic fractures. The majority of these occur in the thoracolumbar region, contributing to the potential development of kyphotic deformities of the spine due to the loss of anterior vertebral body height. More than two-thirds of VCFs are discovered incidentally on diagnostic imaging, suggesting that most of them occur spontaneously with patients unaware of their occurrence or not having clinical symptoms to the extent that they seek medical care. This speaks to the need to consider advanced imaging (magnetic resonance imaging (MRI), computed tomography (CT) or nuclear imaging) in almost all of these patients to clarify the diagnosis.

With the majority of VCFs occurring as a result of osteoporotic fractures, it is important to understand associated risk factors when patients present with a new kyphotic deformity or acute LBP. Osteoporosis is most closely linked to the drop of estrogen after menopause in females with a prevalence of 20% in the United States among postmenopausal women. About 4% of older men will also develop osteoporosis. Other risk factors include genetics, metabolic and endocrine diseases, poor nutrition, low body mass index (BMI), lack of weight-bearing exercise, a sedentary lifestyle, long-term use of glucocorticoids, long-term tobacco and alcohol use, and malignancy. Risk factor mitigation efforts may include nutritional counseling, structured exercise, tobacco and alcohol cessation, the use of calcium and vitamin D supplementation, and—in the case of known osteopenia or osteoporosis—antiresorptive medications, such as bisphosphonates. In young and premenopausal females, family history may play an important role in developing strategies to proactively address modifiable risk factors by maximizing bone mass preservation across the lifespan.

Assessment for a possible VCF generally starts with plain radiographs of the lumbar and/or thoracic spines (see Figure 11.1). As pain from a fracture in the upper lumbar spine may result in pain lower in the back or pelvis, it is important to assess multiple levels above the area of pain. As

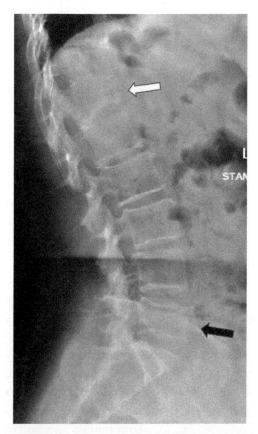

FIGURE 11.1. A standing lateral X-ray showing a compression deformity/fracture of T12 (white arrow). This particularly affects the inferior endplate of the vertebral body. There is also some loss of height of the L5 vertebral body (black arrow). Note that the lumbar X-rays had to be extended into the lower thoracic spine to identify this fracture.

plain radiography has limited sensitivity and cannot necessarily distinguish acute from chronic fractures, nor appropriately assess for underlying malignancy, MRI can be particularly helpful in the evaluation of patients with a suspected acute VCF (see Figure 11.2). MRI is more sensitive in the identification of acute fractures and is superior to plain radiography in assessing for malignancy and neurologic compromise. CT and nuclear imaging may also have a role in certain circumstances. Advanced imaging beyond plain radiography is particularly important to consider in those with a history of cancer, no prior films for comparison, or failure to show improvement.

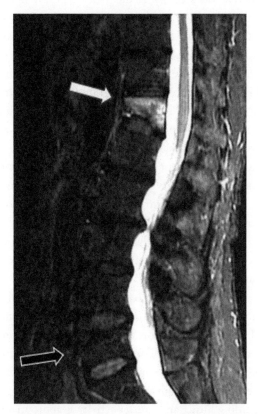

FIGURE 11.2. A sagittal STIR-weighted MRI view of the same patient. Note the bright signal in the T12 vertebral body, consistent with an acute fracture (white arrow). The signal in the L5 vertebral body is normal, suggesting that any alteration in the normal shape of that vertebral body is chronic/longstanding (black arrow).

As the spine is implicated in metastasis in 10–15% of cancers, it is necessary to pursue appropriate diagnostic evaluation in a timely manner when metastasis is suspected. Breast, lung, prostate, and renal cell cancer are particularly associated with spine metastases. As mentioned previously, most cases of VCFs, however, are related to benign osteoporotic fractures. These can generally be managed with a combination of lifestyle modifications and medical therapies to control pain and optimize recovery.

The treatment for acute VCFs centers on patient education and social support, pain control, rehabilitation, and risk factor mitigation. VCFs are stable injuries, meaning that there is usually no need for bracing or surgery to maintain spinal stability. Acute VCFs typically heal on their own with most healing occurring over the first 3 months. Pain, when present, often lasts 4–6 weeks. Patients should be encouraged to walk and move within their tolerance and avoid heavy lifting or high-impact environments. Prolonged bedrest should be avoided, as this may increase the risk of additional VCFs and other complications. Emerging research suggests that patient education and social support may help decrease pain and analgesic requirements and lead to improved mobility and function.

Pain control may be achieved with the judicious use of analgesics. As always, the safest and least restrictive strategies should be employed. In many cases, a combination of acetaminophen and nonsteroidal anti-inflammatory drugs are sufficient to manage acute pain from VCFs, and ongoing research suggest there may be a role for calcitonin for refractory pain control. Opioids are generally not recommended due to insufficient data and concerns about adverse effects including respiratory depression, somnolence, and fall risk.

A rehabilitation strategy should be employed in those with symptomatic VCFs that includes consideration of bracing for short-term care and an exercise-based approach to support a long-term return to premorbid level of function. Bracing with a spinal orthosis such as a lumbar corset or, rarely, a custom-molded brace, may be appropriate for pain control and comfort but is not necessary to maintain stability or improve healing. Some activity restriction regarding lifting and impact activity is appropriate through this time, although walking on land or in a pool, a stationary bike, or other low impact cardiovascular activity should be encouraged. Graded exercise may be supervised or unsupervised, depending on the level of oversight necessary to target the patient's functional goals. Physical therapy for reconditioning and postural stability is often appropriate once pain has been minimized, and there has been time for adequate healing. Importantly for older patients with or at risk of osteoporosis, a focus on balance and coordination to lower the risk of falls should be part of a comprehensive rehabilitation strategy.

Surgical management is typically not indicated in the management of VCFs due to the stable nature of the fracture. A spine surgeon should be consulted if there is neurological dysfunction and/or concern for instability of the spinal column, which is more common in high impact fractures associated with trauma. Current evidence does not support the role of vertebroplasty or kyphoplasty in improving clinical outcomes compared to placebo, and these procedures may be associated with serious adverse events.

The patient in the case presented here experienced acute back pain following a specific inciting event: lifting a heavy object. Her pain is midline and severe, non-radiating and unrelieved by acetaminophen. There is no neurological dysfunction such as motor weakness, numbness, or bowel or bladder dysfunction reported. She has pain with lifting and is having trouble performing activities of daily living (ADLs). Given that she is postmenopausal with risk factors including significant alcohol use during years of maximal bone density, a hysterectomy in her 40s, no resistive exercise regimen and known osteopenia, she is at high risk for a VCF. It is important to pursue imaging upon initial presentation in this case.

The diagnostic evaluation starts with plain radiographs of the lumbar and/or thoracic spine and likely an MRI. MRI should be obtained if the degree of acuity and nature of any fracture identified on plain radiographs is not completely clear or if the radiographs do not show a fracture (Figure 11.2). MRI can also assess for other pathology (such as additional fractures or tumor) and issues in the spinal canal. Were she to have a prior history of cancer, weight loss, malaise, or other risk factors for cancer or fail to improve over the first few weeks of care, an MRI would be essential. For those who cannot have an MRI, a bone scan/nuclear imaging and/or CT should be obtained.

Assuming the imaging shows an acute T12 compression fracture, she should be educated about her fracture, specifically that it is stable, that the pain typically recedes over 6 weeks or so, and that the fracture is most likely going to heal on its own with time. Reassurance may help to lessen fear or anxiety about the nature of the injury. Over the counter analgesics should be optimized. She should be advised to do some light walking on stable surfaces and keep mobile while avoiding any extensive lifting or bending. A cane can be useful early on as can a soft corset for comfort. Topical heat is also reasonable to try. Reclining periodically to relieve pain is also appropriate as long as she is getting up to walk periodically. Home services or enlisting family support may be helpful to assist with meals, cleaning, and other household tasks.

She should be seen again in 2–3 weeks with repeat radiographs to assess for any internal change in the fracture. If doing well and if the fracture is stable, she can then return in 6–8 weeks for another evaluation and repeat X-rays. Physical therapy to help with reconditioning, postural exercise, balance, and home safety should be considered at about 10–12 weeks out from the onset of her fracture.

It is important to recognize that the occurrence of a VCF or other fragility fracture is a defining condition for osteoporosis, independent of prior bone density scores. She should have a comprehensive evaluation and discussion regarding the management of osteoporosis with the intention of minimizing her risk of recurrent fracture.

KEY POINTS

1. VCFs occurs in 25% of females older than 50 years of age and is closely linked to osteoporosis.
2. Most cases of VCFs are asymptomatic or not associated with a specific mechanism of injury.
3. When present, symptoms of VCFs may include moderate to severe pain along the midline of the spine after an injury or activity that exceeds a person's usual level of physical exertion, such as lifting a heavy object.
4. It's important to delineate between a benign and a malignant etiology in the case of VCF for an appropriate care plan.
5. Patient's generally do well with non-interventional care strategies that focus on acute pain control and supportive rehabilitation to promote a return to premorbid levels of function.

Further reading

1. Alsoof D, Anderson G, McDonald CL, Basques B, Kuris E, Daniels AH. Diagnosis and management of vertebral compression fracture. Am J Med. 2022 Mar 17;S0002-9343(22):00192–00199. doi: 10.1016/j.amjmed.2022.02.035. Epub ahead of print. PMID: 35307360.

2. Mauch JT, Carr CM, Cloft H, Diehn FE. Review of the imaging features of benign osteoporotic and malignant vertebral compression fractures. AJNR Am J Neuroradiol. 2018 Sep;39(9):1584–1592. doi: 10.3174/ajnr.A5528. Epub 2018 Jan 18. PMID: 29348133; PMCID: PMC7655272.

3. McCarthy J, Davis A. Diagnosis and management of vertebral compression fractures. Am Fam Physician. 2016 Jul 1;94(1):44–50. PMID: 27386723.

4. Svensson HK, Olsson LE, Hansson T, Karlsson J, Hansson-Olofsson E. The effects of person-centered or other supportive interventions in older women with osteoporotic vertebral compression fractures—a systematic review of the literature. Osteoporos Int. 2017 Jun 6;28(9):2521–2540. PMID: 28585054.

5. Garg B, Dixit V, Batra S, Malhotra R, Sharan A. Non-surgical management of acute osteoporotic vertebral compression fracture: a review. J Clin Orthop Trauma. 2017 Apr-Jun;8(2):131–138. doi: 10.1016/j.jcot.2017.02.001. Epub 2017 Feb 7. PMID: 28720988; PMCID: PMC5498748.

6. Kanchiku T, Taguchi T, Kawai S. Magnetic resonance imaging diagnosis and new classification of the osteoporotic vertebral fracture. J Orthop Sci. 2003;8:463–466. doi: 10.1007/s00776-003-0665-3.

12 "Shouldn't I Be Better by Now?": Persistent Pain after a Compression Fracture

Christopher J. Standaert

This is the patient's third visit for back pain this year.
She is 68 years old and fell 9 months ago. Radiographs
at that time showed a compression fracture at T11
with about 40% loss of vertebral body height. This was
stable on follow-up radiographs 3 months later, at
which point her acute pain had lessened significantly
and she was able to resume walking daily. She is
an accountant but retired several years ago, in part,
to care for her ailing mother. Although she is better
now than shortly after she fell, she complains of
diffuse bilateral pain in her thoracolumbar area and
experiences pain and fatigue if she stands too long.
She went to a few physical therapy visits 6 months
ago and still does some of the stretching exercises
but feels like she is stooped forward when walking.
She has no leg pain. She takes bisphosphonates since
her initial fracture. Radiographs of her thoracic spine
show no changes from 6 months ago, with persistent
wedging of T11 and a healed fracture.

What do you do now?

Although most osteoporotic vertebral compression fractures (VCFs) improve over time, some individuals will have persistent pain and functional limitations. The cause for this is not always clear, but changes in spinal curvature, declines in balance and conditioning, and severity of initial pain may all play a role. It is important to assess posture, physical activity, and barriers to recovery from the initial fracture and to be mindful of the risk of an additional fracture or further injury.

Compression fractures are identified in a large percentage of older women with a prevalence rate of almost 60% in populations of women over 80 years old. Most fractures seem to either occur without symptoms or are not reported to medical providers. The majority of symptomatic VCFs heal over time with significant reduction in symptoms (treatment of acute osteoporotic fractures is discussed in chapter 11). However, about 30–40% of patients will have persistent, significant pain 1 year after a fracture (defined as pain rated >3 on a scale of zero to 10). About 20–25% of individuals will sustain an additional fracture over about 4 years, most of those occurring in the first year after the initial fracture. This rate may be higher in those undergoing vertebral augmentation (kyphoplasty or vertebroplasty). Persistent pain is generally associated with poorer walking capacity, social functioning, mental health, and overall quality of life. Risk factors for persistent pain after a prior VCF are not well identified, but there may be some association with the severity of vertebral body wedging associated with the initial fracture, the initial pain severity, and a lack of regular exercise prior to sustaining a fracture. In general, osteoporotic women identified with a VCF have higher levels of back pain compared to those without VCFs.

The etiology of persistent pain after a VCF is not clear. Assuming the bone heals, that would not seem a common source of pain. In thinking through the consequences of an acute, symptomatic VCF, there are several potential reasons why some may have persistent pain. These include the acute consequences on their physical function, general health, and psychological health. They also include structural changes to the spine that tend to increase thoracic kyphosis (the anterior curvature of the thoracic spine). Addressing some of these factors, ideally in the course of acute treatment, or later once the acute injury has healed, can help improve pain and function.

The acute treatment of a VCF generally involves relative rest or activity restriction, medications for pain, and potentially bracing or interventional procedures. All of these can have consequences for affected individuals. Bed rest in older adults results in dramatic reductions in lean muscle mass and strength. Declines in balance and increases in fall risk are seen in those with compression fractures. About 3% of patients with an acute VCF will have a major medical complication within the first 30 days after their fracture, pulmonary function declines in those with chronic obstructive pulmonary disease following a VCF, and about half of patients sustaining a VCF will receive opiates acutely. There has been limited research into the psychological response to a VCF, but the existing literature supports concern for increased depression, anxiety, and fear. Fear alone may encompass several domains, including fear of falling, fear of pain, and fear of isolation. All of these psychological or mental health states seem potentially amenable to structured treatment in patients with a VCF.

An important component of persistent pain following a VCF is the effect on spinal alignment, particularly an increase in thoracic kyphosis. VCFs typically involve a wedge-shaped fracture, with the anterior portion of the vertebral body collapsing more than the posterior portion. This increases the anterior tilt of the spine at that level, hence a thoracic VCF typically increases the thoracic kyphosis or anterior angulation of the thoracic spine (see Figure 12.1). Increasing the thoracic kyphosis, in turn, may cause a new (or enhance a preexisting) sagittal imbalance of the spine, which has significant functional consequences. Ideally, the lordotic/posterior curve of the lumbar spine is in balance with the kyphotic/anterior curve of the thoracic spine, keeping the center of mass of the torso balanced over the middle of the pelvis. Sagittal imbalance refers to a condition where this is not the case, and the center of mass is either posterior to the middle of the . pelvis (negative sagittal imbalance) or anterior to the middle of the pelvis (positive sagittal imbalance), making it difficult to balance while standing. Hyperkyphosis of the thoracic spine (defined as a curvature of greater than 40°), often associated with a VCF, results in a positive sagittal imbalance.

Thoracic hyperkyphosis occurs in about 20% or older women and is clearly associated with VCFs. This has a host of negative consequences, including reduced balance, back pain, increased fall risk, reduction in health-related quality of life, difficulty performing activities of daily living (ADLs), reduced walking speed, increased truncal sway with walking, increased fatigue, and higher mortality rates. This can also negatively impact self-image

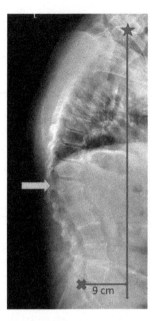

FIGURE 12.1. A lateral standing radiograph (sagittal plane) showing a chronic wedge-shaped compression fracture at T12 (arrow) with a subsequent kyphosis at this level. Note that the thoracic spine angles forward above the fracture. The vertical line drawn down from the middle of the C7 vertebrae (star) should pass through the posterior aspect of S1 (X). In this case, the increase in kyphosis from the fracture causes the line from C7 to pass 9 cm anteriorly to the posterior aspect of S1. This is termed a positive sagittal imbalance.

and social interaction and can increase the fear of falling. It is commonly thought to also be associated with muscular weakness or sarcopenia (loss of muscle cells) in the paraspinal musculature. There are a number of studies assessing treatment and, particularly, the effects of exercise for thoracic hyperkyphosis and sagittal imbalance. Exercise that includes work on trunk flexibility, spinal extensor strengthening, balance, and respiratory muscles while avoiding spinal/trunk flexion (such as abdominal crunches) seems to be particularly helpful in addressing function, pain, posture, and potential risk of subsequent fracture. The exercise programs shown to be beneficial are generally relatively long-term, meaning up to 6 to 12 months and likely should be performed indefinitely by patients with hyperkyphosis. Several visits to physical therapy early after a fracture are not adequate. Clearly optimizing the management of osteoporosis may be helpful in maintaining the long-term health of those with hyperkyphosis by reducing the risk of additional fractures. Bracing may have a role symptomatically, but brace use should be balanced with exercise so as not to promote further weakness or loss of spinal mobility.

In considering the patient presented above, we can begin to see how to understand her situation and help her. She sustained a fall, which deserves more exploration. Defining her fall risks, be they issues in the home or community or structural/physiologic issues related to her spine, balance, neurologic function, and strength is important. It is worth discussing how and why she fell in the first place. It is helpful to explore her recovery, any change from her baseline activities, exercise, or ADLs since her fracture, and how she manages her pain. One might predict that she is at a lower functional level than she was and likely only utilizes passive approaches to her pain like rest and over the counter medication. It is critical to understand her interest in and barriers to exercise, as this will be an essential part of her treatment. She will need to recognize the importance of this in maintaining her health and function and addressing her pain. Assessing fear, anxiety, and depression will be helpful in recognizing their potential contribution to her current state. Nutritional status and weight gain or weight loss also play a role in her rehabilitation.

Physical examination should include palpation of her spine for tenderness, inspection for hyperkyphosis, sagittal imbalance, and a potential associated scoliosis. Trunk range of motion into flexion and extension and hip range of motion should be assessed. Gait, balance, lower extremity strength, and neurologic function, including vibration and/or proprioception, are all important in understanding her functional capacity, fall risk, and rehabilitation needs. Given that she is at risk for sustaining another fracture, it would be appropriate to obtain standing lumbar spine X-rays and full length standing scoliosis X-rays to assess her sagittal balance (scoliosis and scoliosis X-rays are discussed in chapter 10). Assuming these show no further fractures or related concerns, there is likely no added benefit to further imaging, given the absence of any neurologic symptoms or findings.

Treatment should center around an exercise-based approach that focuses on spinal extension, gait, balance, range of motion, respiratory function, and fall prevention. These are generally best addressed by a comprehensive physical therapy program with ongoing independent participation in exercise. She currently walks some, but that is not adequate to maintain her spine. Adaptive devices like canes, walking sticks, or walkers may offer substantial benefit for ambulation if she has a significant positive sagittal imbalance. Occupational therapy may be helpful in optimizing her function at home, including basic house chores, her kitchen layout, and routine ADLs. She may benefit from home care or other assistance for heavy lifting or tasks that require trunk flexion or high loads on her spine. Depending upon her psychological functioning, she may benefit from work with a psychologist on coping and adaptation to the changes in her spine. Addressing fear, anxiety, depression, and negative self-image may all improve her well-being and long-term health. Bracing, usually a soft corset, can be considered for periodic symptomatic relief or to enhance her ability to stand for any extended period. Medications should generally be restricted to over the counter analgesics. Opiates have no evidence of benefit here and could be very problematic. Her bone density should be addressed appropriately. With a stable, healed fracture, there is no role for vertebral augmentation like vertebroplasty or kyphoplasty. Without neurologic concerns, progressive postural decline, or marked functional impairment associated with her fracture and spinal deformity, there is likely no role for surgical care. By helping her understand her spine and providing her with a comprehensive approach to function better and live more effectively, there is potential to substantially improve her life.

KEY POINTS

1. 30–40% of patients sustaining a painful, acute VCF will have at least mild to moderate pain 1 year later.
2. About 25% of those who sustain an initial acute VCF will sustain an additional fracture in the next 4 years.
3. Hyperkyphosis associated with increased vertebral wedging from a fracture can have substantial negative consequences on activity and health.
4. Exercise focusing on spinal extension, gait, balance, range of motion, respiratory function, and fall prevention is critical in the management of pain following a VCF.

5. Depression, isolation, fear of falling or further injury, and negative self-image may all be persistent consequences of a VCF and can be addressed therapeutically.

Further reading

1. Cui L, Chen L, Xia W, et al. Vertebral fracture in postmenopausal Chinese women: a population-based study. Osteoporos Int. 2017 Sep;28(9):2583–2590. doi: 10.1007/s00198-017-4085-1. Epub 2017 May 30. PMID: 28560474.

2. Gold LS, O'Reilly MK, Heagerty PJ, Jarvik JG. Complications and healthcare utilization in commercially-insured osteoporotic vertebral compression fracture patients: a comparison of kyphoplasty versus propensity-matched controls. Spine J. 2021 Aug;21(8):1347–1354. doi: 10.1016/j.spinee.2021.03.025. Epub 2021 Mar 26. PMID: 33781968; PMCID: PMC8349787.

3. Katzman WB, Wanek L, Shepherd JA, Sellmeyer DE. Age-related hyperkyphosis: its causes, consequences, and management. J Orthop Sports Phys Ther. 2010 Jun;40(6):352–360. doi: 10.2519/jospt.2010.3099. PMID: 20511692; PMCID: PMC2907357.

4. Kortebein P, Ferrando A, Lombeida J, Wolfe R, Evans WJ. Effect of 10 days of bed rest on skeletal muscle in healthy older adults. JAMA. 2007 Apr 25;297(16):1772–1774. doi: 10.1001/jama.297.16.1772-b. PMID: 17456818.

5. Venmans A, Klazen CA, Lohle PN, Mali WP, van Rooij WJ. Natural history of pain in patients with conservatively treated osteoporotic vertebral compression fractures: results from VERTOS II. AJNR Am J Neuroradiol. 2012 Mar;33(3):519–521. doi: 10.3174/ajnr.A2817. Epub 2011 Nov 24. PMID: 22116114; PMCID: PMC7966424.

13 "I Fell Off a Ladder, and My Back Really Hurts.": Acute Trauma in a 38-Year-Old Male

Anthony A. Oyekan, Dominic Ridolfi, Christopher Gibbs, Jeremy D. Shaw

A 38-year-old male presents with 2 days of severe upper lumbar pain. He states he was getting on a ladder while painting the exterior of his house when he fell, dropping about 4 feet onto his backside. He had immediate pain in his upper lumbar area that has not gone away. He has been able to walk and has had no leg symptoms, but it hurts to stand and be vertical in general. He is healthy otherwise with no ongoing medical problems. He does not smoke and drinks about 3 alcoholic beverages per week. He plays soccer regularly, likes to camp, and is generally active overall.

What do you do now?

Vertebral burst fractures are common injuries in high-energy mechanisms, such as high falls. Common presentations include severe axial back pain, radicular leg symptoms, or neurological deficits. A burst fracture, not to be confused with a compression fracture, is a severe injury that may require acute operative intervention. A thorough history and physical examination, appropriate imaging, accurate diagnosis, and appropriate treatment plan will improve the recovery rate and quality.

Thoracolumbar fractures are best understood using the three-column concept—a system developed by Dr. Francis Denis in 1983 that remains central to modern classification systems. Here, the spine has three parallel columns—anterior, middle, and posterior—along with their respective anatomical elements. The anterior column consists of the anterior longitudinal ligament (ALL), anterior two-thirds of the vertebral body, and anterior two-thirds of the intervertebral disc (see Figure 13.1). Similarly, the middle column consists of the posterior longitudinal ligament (PLL) and the posterior one-third of the vertebral body and intervertebral disc. The posterior column consists of all structures posterior to the PLL: the posterior bony arch—including the pedicles and lamina—and the posterior ligamentous complex (PLC)—including the supraspinous ligament, interspinous ligament, capsule, and ligamentum flavum. The middle column and the PLC are the most critical structures to spinal stability. Three-column injuries represent the most severe spinal injuries in contrast to less severe single-column involvement.

The three-column concept also helps to describe the injury morphology of burst and compression fractures. While both fracture types are due to axial loading, compression fractures are generally lower energy and may have an anterior flexion moment, leading to the anterior column's failure. Burst fractures, in contrast, are higher energy injuries caused by pure axial compression wherein both the anterior and middle columns are injured. As the middle column is involved in a burst fracture, the fracture extends into the posterior aspect of the vertebral body adjacent to the spinal canal. Injury to the middle column may cause bony retropulsion of bone—displacement of bone from the vertebral body into the spinal canal—which can cause spinal stenosis and associated neurological deficits.

It is essential to recognize that spinal fractures don't always fall into classically described categories, and there is a spectrum of severity for

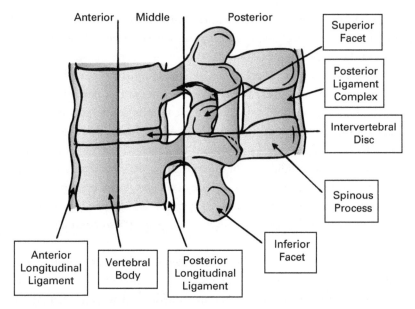

Anterior   Middle   Posterior

Superior
Facet

Posterior
Ligament
Complex

Intervertebral
Disc

Spinous
Process

Inferior
Facet

Anterior
Longitudinal
Ligament

Vertebral
Body

Posterior
Longitudinal
Ligament

FIGURE 13.1. The Denis 3 columns of the spine. Anterior column (dark gray): Anterior Longitudinal Ligament (ALL), anterior 2/3 vertebral body, and anterior intervertebral disc. Middle column (gray): posterior 1/3 vertebral body, posterior intervertebral disc, and posterior longitudinal ligament (PLL). Posterior column (light gray): all structures posterior to the PLL.

these injuries. For instance, some burst fractures are stable and treated nonoperatively, while unstable ones may require surgical intervention. In burst fractures with the extension of the damage into the bony or ligamentous posterior column and therefore greater instability, surgical management is more likely. The key takeaway is that burst fractures are higher energy injuries that are less stable than compression fractures.

The thoracolumbar region accounts for 90% of spinal fractures, with burst fractures presenting the most common unstable fracture pattern. As above, this pattern comes from high-energy and axial-loaded mechanisms of injury, such as a high fall, motorcycle accident, or high-impact sports. Given the nature of these mechanisms, it's common for patients to present with multiple injuries, such as long bone fractures, chest/abdominal trauma, and other spinal fractures. Notably, 10% of patients with a thoracolumbar burst fracture have at least one other burst fracture from the exact same injury, 53% of which are at noncontiguous levels. To further emphasize the importance of comprehensive examination, over 25% of patients with thoracolumbar fractures also have distant spine fractures, often in the cervical spine.

In this case, the patient presents with upper lumbar pain, without lower extremity symptoms, 2 days following the injury. The next critical step is neurological evaluation, as deficits are common in patients with burst fractures (up to 30%) and indicate the need for magnetic resonance imaging (MRI) and surgical intervention. By contrast, neurologically intact patients may be candidates for nonoperative management. Symptoms indicating a neurological deficit include new onset, lower extremity motor weakness, sensory loss, radicular pain, paresthesia, saddle anesthesia, and bowel or bladder dysfunction. Severe back pain is also common, as expected with a fracture.

Physical examination findings in patients with burst fractures vary but may include localized tenderness, crepitus, abrasions, or ecchymosis. Neurologic examination checklists are beneficial. The American Spinal Cord Injury Association (ASIA) impairment scale (AIS) is a readily available example. Examine patients for motor function, sensory function, and reflexes. In addition, a genitourinary exam, including rectal tone and perianal sensation, should be performed in patients with suspected conus medullaris syndrome or cauda equina syndrome. Bear in mind that significant pain may limit examination and lead to missed neurological deficits. Nevertheless, any neurological deficit should be considered a red flag that warrants urgent attention until proven otherwise.

There are several imaging studies of relevance in patients with burst fractures. If the patient in the case example presented to an outpatient office, the initial imaging study of choice is plain radiographs. Radiographs to order include anterior-posterior (AP), lateral, and possible flexion/extension views of the lumbar spine. Physicians should also image the cervical and thoracic spine with AP and lateral radiographs. Recall that concomitant spinal fractures are common. Findings on AP X-rays may include widened space between pedicles or coronal plane deformity at the fracture level. The lateral view may show a sagittal plane deformity, including kyphosis or retropulsion. Note that plain films may not show the true extent of injury, such as bony retropulsion. Flexion/extension views may show increased gapping between spinous processes with flexion, indicating a ligamentous posterior column injury. Still, patients may not move adequately on these views due to pain. Plain films are generally not needed in trauma centers as computed tomography (CT) scans are routinely obtained and allow greater sensitivity in detecting burst fractures. Order a CT scan of the spine for all patients with a burst fracture identified on plain films after acute injury; contrast is unnecessary (see Figure 13.2).

Imaging should evaluate several vertebral levels above and below the identified or suspected injury to facilitate morphological assessment and operative planning. A non-contrast thoracic and lumbar CT scan is appropriate. If full-spine radiographs are unavailable, proceed with a CT scan of the entire spine (cervical, thoracic, lumbar). Order non-contrast MRI in the event of neurological deficits or unclear injury to the PLC (on flexion radiographs or CT) given a superior evaluation of spinal cord or thecal sac compression. It is worth contacting an Orthopedic Surgery or Neurosurgery consultant in this case, as these patients often require surgery and transfer to a higher level of care. MRIs evaluate for hematoma, ligamentous injury, and spinal cord edema. CT myelogram is an appropriate alternative for patients with MRI-incompatible devices, including pacemakers.

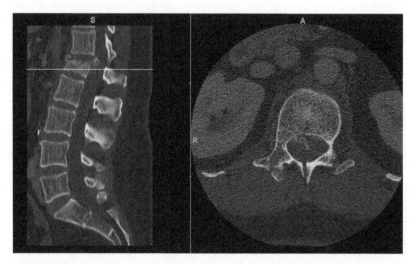

FIGURE 13.2. Sagittal (left) and axial (right) imaging of an L1 burst fracture with retropulsion and kyphotic deformity. Note the fracture extension to the posterior vertebral body with fragment retropulsion into the spinal canal and associated lamina fracture.

Treatment of burst fractures is multifactorial and considers the patient's physiologic age/function, neurologic status, fracture pattern, ligamentous injury, deformity, and associated injuries. The Thoracolumbar Injury Classification and Severity (TLICS) scale is a commonly used classification system, which focuses on fracture morphology (CT scan), neurological status, and PLC integrity (CT or MRI) to guide treatment. Scores of 3 or lower indicate nonoperative management; scores of 5 or greater indicate operative management; and a score of 4 indicates equipoise between operative or nonoperative management at the treating surgeon's discretion. For example, a neurologically intact patient with an isolated burst fracture and no ligamentous injury would have a TLICS score of 2 and be a candidate for nonoperative management—e.g. activity as tolerated and a thoracolumbosacral orthosis (TLSO) for comfort. In contrast, a patient with a lumbar burst fracture, PLC injury, and L1 nerve root deficit (e.g. hip flexion weakness or groin radicular sensory change) would have a TLICS score of 7 and be a candidate for operative intervention (e.g. neurologic decompression with spinal stabilization). Aside from TLICS, other indications for operative management include neurologic deficits with radiographic evidence of compression, PLC injury, progressive kyphosis, uncontrolled pain with inability to mobilize, and polytrauma. Although the patient in our case study had a late presentation, he may be a candidate for surgery regardless of neurological status or extent of retropulsion if he has a burst fracture with PLC injury.

Outcomes for operative vs. nonoperative management of stable fractures in neurologically intact patients are presently considered equivalent. However, clear indications for surgery do exist. Bracing is useful primarily for symptomatic relief—TLSO braces have not been shown to improve outcomes and can be uncomfortable. Physicians should not use prolonged bed rest to treat any spine fracture. Prolonged bed rest is associated with numerous complications, including increased risk of deep venous thromboembolism, pulmonary embolus, and pneumonia. Physicians should follow recommendations from spine surgeons to resume activity as tolerated. Patients with neurological deficits or unstable injuries require operative intervention. However, surgery is not without the risk of complication.

Complications include surgical site infection, incidental durotomy, iatrogenic nerve injury, ileus, or mechanical complications. Some complications may require reoperation.

Refer every burst fracture to a spine specialist. Although every burst fracture doesn't need surgery, even "stable" fractures may require serial radiographs for as long as 3 to 6 months.

KEY POINTS

1. A burst fracture is differentiated from a compression fracture by the involvement of the middle column of the spine (fracture extension to the posterior vertebral body).
2. Always evaluate for concomitant noncontiguous spine injuries, as 10% of patients with a burst fracture have multiple burst fractures.
3. Burst fractures are severe injuries; 30% of patients present with a neurological deficit.
4. Plain film radiographs (X-rays) are an appropriate initial imaging study in a patient with a suspected burst fracture presenting to an ambulatory clinic; follow-up CT or MRI is often indicated.
5. Burst fractures should be referred to a spine specialist.

Further reading

1. Wood KB, Buttermann GR, Phukan R, et al. Operative compared with nonoperative treatment of a thoracolumbar burst fracture without neurological deficit: a prospective randomized study with follow-up at sixteen to twenty-two years. J Bone Joint Surg Am. 2015 Jan 7;97(1):3–9. doi: 10.2106/JBJS.N.00226. PMID: 25568388.
2. Scheer JK, Bakhsheshian J, Fakurnejad S, Oh T, Dahdaleh NS, Smith ZA. Evidence-based medicine of traumatic thoracolumbar burst fractures: a systematic review of operative management across 20 years. Global Spine J. 2015 Feb;5(1):73–82. doi: 10.1055/s-0034-1396047. Epub 2014 Nov 24. PMID: 25648401; PMCID: PMC4303483.

3. Bailey CS, Dvorak MF, Thomas KC, et al. Comparison of thoracolumbosacral orthosis and no orthosis for the treatment of thoracolumbar burst fractures: interim analysis of a multicenter randomized clinical equivalence trial. J Neurosurg Spine. 2009 Sep;11(3):295–303. doi: 10.3171/2009.3.SPINE08312. PMID: 19769510.
4. Denis F. Spinal instability as defined by the three-column spine concept in acute spinal trauma. Clin Orthop Relat Res. 1984 Oct;(189):65–76. PMID: 6478705.
5. Lee JY, Vaccaro AR, Lim MR, et al. Thoracolumbar injury classification and severity score: a new paradigm for the treatment of thoracolumbar spine trauma. J Orthop Sci. 2005 Nov;10(6):671–675. doi: 10.1007/s00776-005-0956-y. PMID: 16307197; PMCID: PMC2779435.

14 "I've Been Coughing a Lot, Too.": A 68-Year-Old Smoker with a Cough and Back Pain

Robert L. Bailey, Jessica Sullivan

A patient that you have known for many years comes in with a new symptom of back pain. He has known COPD with a long history of smoking, although he stopped smoking several years ago. He also had a cardiac stent placed last year. He lives by himself and continues to work doing minor home repairs. He does not exercise otherwise and is sedentary at home. With his pulmonary disease, he notes a chronic cough and intermittent shortness of breath that has been more problematic lately. Over the last year or so, he has noted pain involving his low thoracic to upper lumbar area. This is worse with standing compared to sitting, but also awakens him from sleep at night. He notes some degree of depression recently along with a decreased appetite. He has lost about 8 pounds in the past 6 months that he attributes to the change in appetite. On exam, he is a thin male who stoops forward mildly when standing. He is not tender in his spine and has normal strength and reflexes in his legs.

What do you do now?

When patients present with new onset pain, consider specific factors regarding severity, frequency, timing, location, and distribution. If the patient is known to you, changes in these variables will help guide an appropriate investigation. Several aspects of this patient's presentation are worrisome, including his history of smoking, pain awakening him at night, and loss of weight. These all might suggest an underlying neoplasm, most specifically lung cancer. Hopefully, the patient has already completed Low Dose CT scan per United States Preventive Services Task Force (USPTF) criteria, to screen for early signs of malignant nodules. Screening for a family history of breast cancer and personal history of prostate cancer should be included in his evaluation. Essentially all cancers carry a risk of metastases to the spine, but the most common to occur are lung, breast, prostate, renal cell, myeloma, lymphoma, thyroid, and melanoma.

The type of pain associated with spinal metastases can be further delineated by local, radicular, and mechanical features. Localization of pain can pinpoint the initial diagnostic imaging needed. Pain can be radicular in nature, and close attention to the distribution is required, as it relates to dermatomes in cervical, thoracic, and lumbar regions. Mechanical pain could be worsened by movements such as neck flexion, straight-leg-raise, sneezing, coughing, or straining. Characteristically, patients with epidural metastases will frequently experience pain that persists in recumbency, especially at night. Some will have associated numbness, tingling, and/or stiffness.

Tumor, either primary or metastatic, is one of the "red flag" conditions in spine care, along with fracture, infection, and cauda equina or other severe neurological compromise. A history of cancer is the factor most strongly associated with spinal tumor, with age >50 or <20 years old, night pain, and constitutional symptoms (like weight loss) also being relevant. In the setting of suspected cancer, it is important to identify the presence of weakness, balance loss, and bowel or bladder changes. Neurogenic bowel and bladder changes may entail urinary retention or bowel and/or bladder incontinence where there is no sensation of either movement. Stress or urge incontinence at times will overlap the true incontinence and should be carefully teased out during the interview. For instance, did the patient feel the process of voiding or having a bowel movement vs. no sensation at all?

These symptoms all suggest involvement of the spinal cord, cauda equina, or individual nerve roots.

On physical examination, the patient should have good resistance to strength testing in their arms and legs. If they have significant change in gait disturbances, more than their baseline, there should be concern of a myelopathic process. Myelopathy is a spinal cord injury secondary to compressive pathology. Tumors and disc herniations are major contributors to myelopathy, along with traumatic injuries to bone and/or ligaments.

The following muscle groups should be tested to determine myotomal deficits pertaining to certain nerve root(s) involvement.

Upper extremities: deltoids (shoulder abduction), biceps (elbow flexion), triceps (elbow extension), finger flexors (grip), and hand intrinsics (finger extension/abduction).

Lower extremities: iliopsoas (hip flexors), quadriceps (knee extension), anterior tibialis (foot dorsiflexion), gastrocnemius (foot plantar flexion), and extensor hallucis longus (big toe extension).

For this gentleman with a significant smoking history and new onset of back pain as well as associated cough and unintentional weight loss, plain radiographs and magnetic resonance imaging (MRI) of the thoracic and lumbar spines with and without intravenous contrast is indicated. When concern for malignancy exists, ordering an MRI to include post contrast images is most appropriate to better allow for the identification of soft tissue or bony lesions. If MRI imaging is consistent with tumor, computed tomography (CT) scans of the chest, abdomen, and pelvis are necessary to determine systemic tumor burden and assess for a primary cancer site. A bone scan will also be helpful to look for other skeletal lesions. Few lesions in the spine are primary in origin, and, more commonly, there is high suspicion for systemic metastases.

Once a spinal lesion is discovered, a spine surgeon will evaluate for degree of involvement of the bone, epidural extension of the tumor, and compression of spinal cord or thecal sac. Depending on those imaging characteristics, this will guide recommendations as to whether the patient should proceed first with spine surgery or if, instead, it would be worthwhile to obtain a biopsy of the lesion at the site of origin (e.g. lung biopsy). Biopsy of a primary tumor outside of the spine may be less invasive, and pathology may dictate oncological and surgical management. In some cases, surgery would not be necessary. Consultation with medical oncology and possibly radiation oncology at this time will also be beneficial to coordinate decision-making with the patient and treatment teams.

When tumor infiltrates the spine, it may result in pathological fracture of the vertebral body and subsequent structural instability. The thoracolumbar injury classification and severity (TLICS) score is a common algorithm that is used to assist the surgeon in the management of an oncological patient. This algorithm guides the decision as to whether a patient would benefit from surgical intervention and determines the need for structural stabilization. Management based on a TLICS score of <3 is considered nonoperative, 4 is a "grey zone" and can be operative or nonoperative, and >5 is operative. Characteristics such as burst compression fracture with neurological deficits are likely to lead to consideration for surgery, whereas a pathological compression fracture without neurological deficits or instability may be more amenable to nonsurgical treatment. The details of algorithms are not important for nonsurgical clinicians to know, but they do help illustrate the recommendation that the patient be seen by an experienced spine surgeon for detailed analysis of the varying radiographic findings and clinical presentation to determine the role for surgery in the context of the overall treatment goals of the patient and care team.

Not all metastatic lesions will require surgical intervention, and many of these patients can be managed within the outpatient setting. The evaluation of a patient for concern of oncological metastases to the spine is of an urgent nature. However, some symptoms need to be evaluated on an emergent basis in an effort to avoid permanent loss of neurological function. The following is a list of broad criteria for when a patient with known or suspected spinal metastases should be referred to the emergency department for timely diagnostic workup and evaluation.

- o Acute weakness: when a patient cannot resist on strength testing exam or walk without assistance due to their legs giving out (as opposed to subjective weakness limited by pain)
- o Cauda equina symptoms: including saddle anesthesia, urinary retention, urinary/fecal incontinence, reduced anal sphincter tone, acute sexual dysfunction, and significant motor weakness that

may or may not be associated with low back pain or radicular pain (sciatica)

o Acute loss of sensation in a specific dermatome—for this case, thoracic, lumbar, and saddle regions should be tested

o Extensive lesions and infiltration on imaging

If performed, the goal of surgery should be to preserve or restore neurological function, as well as to decompress and stabilize the spine. For some cases, the prognosis and staging of the cancer would impact the decision to undergo surgical intervention. If patients have a prognosis of less than 3–4 months, surgery may not be the best option, as their postoperative course may consume the remainder of their lifespan with expected surgical pain and activity restrictions. Patients should have an informed discussion with the palliative care and oncology teams along with the spine surgeon on anticipated outcome and expectations from surgical intervention.

Nonsurgical management, that is, chemotherapy and radiation therapy, is preferable to surgery in certain diagnostic instances. As an example, primary diagnoses such as myeloma and lymphoma are considered radiosensitive tumors. Depending on imaging characteristics, neurologic status, and systemic disease, the patient may be recommended for palliative radiation to the spine lesion to shrink the size of the tumor rather than surgical decompression and excision. Radiation therapy can also routinely be scheduled to follow surgery to adequately address the residual tumor or tumor bed post resection, which has been shown to improve pain, tumor control, and neurologic deficits. Not many tumors can be resected in their entirety without causing iatrogenic neurologic deficits, so postoperative radiation therapy is typically required for completeness of treatment. Timing of radiation should be coordinated with the surgical team to ensure complete wound healing, as the risk of wound breakdown and dehiscence from radiation is greatly increased.

Back pain is one of the most common symptoms for patients seen in the primary care setting. The importance of screening the past medical and family history along with obtaining diagnostic testing will help capture accurate diagnoses and lead to appropriate referral to specialties when suspicion for malignancy arises.

1. Tumor represents one of the "red flag" conditions in spine management and should be considered in every patient presenting with acute, progressive, or persistent symptoms.
2. A history of cancer is the factor most strongly associated with spinal tumor for ages >50 or <20 years old, with night pain and constitutional symptoms (like weight loss) also being relevant.
3. When patients at high risk for cancer present with acute weakness or other neurologic concerns, it is best to direct them to the emergency department for urgent evaluation and imaging.
4. In the setting of spinal metastases, surgical vs. nonsurgical management decision-making is multifactorial and based on patient's imaging, neurological status, prognosis, preferences, and if available, tumor diagnosis.
5. Patients with spinal tumors require a multidisciplinary approach. This is an emotionally taxing and stressful diagnosis for the patient and their families. However, the primary care provider can be the one familiar voice to help patients understand their diagnosis and treatment options along with the surgical and oncological teams.

Further reading

1. Greenberg MS. "Spinal Epidural Metastases." In *Handbook of Neurosurgery*, 8th ed., 814–822. New York: Thieme, 2020.
2. Sciubba DM, Petteys RJ, Dekutoski MB, et al. Diagnosis and management of metastatic spine disease: A Review. J Neurosurg Spine. 2010;13(1):94–108. doi: 10.3171/2010.3.SPINE09202.
3. Spratt DE, Beeler WH, Moraes FY, et al. An integrated multidisciplinary algorithm for the management of spinal metastases: an International Spine Oncology Consortium report. Lancet Oncol. 2017;13(12): e720–e730. doi: 10.1016/S1470-2045(17)30612-5.

15 "My Lungs Are Better, but Now My Back Hurts.": Back Pain after Pneumonia

Joseph P. Shivers, Christopher J. Standaert

A 45-year-old man comes to see you for recent onset low back pain (LBP). He was in the hospital with an acute bacterial pneumonia just last month and had no pain at that time. He notes some minor transient episodes of LBP in the past, but they have been mild and self-limiting. His current pain has been progressively increasing since he was discharged from the hospital. He completed his antibiotics shortly after discharge. He is on a tumor necrosis factor (TNF)-alpha inhibitor for inflammatory bowel disease, and that condition has been stable for several years. He thought he was getting better after his pneumonia but feels like he is still fatigued. He had no new injury and is really not back to the same level of activity that he had before the pneumonia. Over the counter analgesics and stretching at home have not been helping his pain, which radiates across his low back and is constant.

What do you do now?

This patient's case includes several troubling elements. In contrast to his previous mild self-limited back pain, now his LBP is actually worsening with time. He cannot find a position of comfort. He is immunosuppressed at baseline, he had a recent bacterial infection which immediately preceded the onset of back pain, and his symptoms include fatigue. These factors are concerning for the possibility of an infection, specifically vertebral osteomyelitis.

Osteomyelitis is an infection of bone, from the Greek osteo (bone) + myelo (marrow) + itis (inflammation). Vertebral osteomyelitis, also known as spondylodiscitis or septic discitis, is an infection of the vertebral column. If the infection arrives via the bloodstream (hematogenously), it typically starts at a vertebral endplate, which is the layer of cartilage at the top or bottom of each vertebral body that bounds the upper or lower portion, respectively, of the intervertebral disc. Infection then spreads from the endplate to the adjacent disc, which is avascular. Alternatively, vertebral osteomyelitis can arise by local spread (e.g. from nearby abscess, in the course of a traumatic injury, or during a medical procedure).

Vertebral osteomyelitis is sometimes classified, based on causative organism, as pyogenic (e.g. *Staph. aureus*, *E. coli*), non-pyogenic (tuberculosis or brucellosis), or fungal (e.g. *Candida*). Risk factors for brucellosis and tuberculosis include a relatively indolent clinical course and a history of residence or travel in an endemic area. Risk factors for fungal infection include significant immunocompromise, history of intravenous drug use, and indwelling intravenous catheters. In clinical practice, non-pyogenic, and fungal causes should be considered especially if bacterial cultures are not growing an organism.

Most patients with vertebral osteomyelitis present with pain of the low back, upper back, or neck, depending on where the infection is. Pyogenic vertebral osteomyelitis is seen most commonly in the lumbar spine, whereas tuberculosis tends to infect the thoracic spine. Almost half of patients with vertebral osteomyelitis are afebrile at the time of presentation, possibly because many patients take over the counter pain relievers which can mask fever. Most patients do not have any neurologic symptoms.

Because vertebral osteomyelitis is rare and its symptoms are nonspecific, diagnosis is often delayed. Analogously to cancer, infection must be considered in every patient who presents with back or neck pain. Risk factors for vertebral osteomyelitis include intravenous drug use, diabetes mellitus, immunosuppression, rheumatic disease, alcoholism, liver failure, and renal failure. Known preceding bacterial infection is certainly of concern, though an initial source ends up being identified in only half of vertebral osteomyelitis cases. Patients should be asked about red-flag symptoms such as new or progressive weakness or numbness, gait imbalance, and bowel or bladder incontinence.

Physical exam should include vital signs (fever and hemodynamic instability are concerning), palpation over the site of pain (severe vertebral-column tenderness is concerning), and neurologic evaluation with attention to gait, sensation, strength, and reflexes (the presence of any neurologic deficit in spine infection is highly concerning for associated spinal epidural abscess, which can progress to cause paralysis and incontinence). Although the physical exam can elevate the level of concern and might even reveal an emergency (e.g. sepsis, polyradiculopathy), an unremarkable physical exam does not rule out the possibility of vertebral osteomyelitis.

The best-validated screening blood tests are erythrocyte sedimentation rate (ESR) and C-reactive protein (CRP). Elevation in either ESR or CRP has a sensitivity of 94–100% for vertebral osteomyelitis, so these tests in combination are helpful to rule out the condition. By contrast, white blood cell (WBC) count is often normal or only mildly elevated in vertebral osteomyelitis.

The lab workup for possible vertebral osteomyelitis is also recommended to include two sets of blood cultures, with each set targeting both anaerobic and aerobic organisms. In the outpatient setting, if our clinical concern is relatively low, we typically start with ESR and CRP only, and if these are both negative, then we do not routinely obtain blood cultures.

The preferred diagnostic imaging modality is magnetic resonance imaging (MRI), which is highly sensitive and specific. The use of intravenous (IV) gadolinium contrast is recommended as a way to increase both specificity and sensitivity of MRI. Given the risks of gadolinium toxicity in patients with impaired renal function, creatinine should be considered as part of the initial lab workup if the patient's kidney function hasn't already recently been tested. Early in the course of infection, MRI results can be inconclusive; in the event of ongoing clinical concern without definitive imaging, a repeat MRI 1–2 weeks later can be helpful, as the findings on

MRI generally progress with time. If MRI is not feasible, strong alternative options include nuclear imaging with single-photon emission computed tomography (SPECT) using a combination of Technetium-99m and Gallium-67, or positron emission tomography/computed tomography (PET/CT). Even conventional computed tomography (CT) of the lumbar spine has fairly good sensitivity (84–100%). Plain radiographs are easy to obtain and are routinely performed as part of the workup for concerning LBP. Erosive or destructive changes in the vertebral body endplates can appear within weeks of an infection, but early on, these findings may be subtle, so it is important to know that radiographs are not highly sensitive for vertebral osteomyelitis (i.e. they cannot rule out the disease).

For the outpatient clinician, the most important things about vertebral osteomyelitis are to consider the diagnosis and, if warranted, to test for it. In a patient with known intravenous drug use who comes to the office with a fever and tachycardia, the correct next step is transfer to the emergency department. In a patient whose chronic axial LBP seems vaguely different and worse than usual and has risk factors for infection, the next step is to order ESR and CRP. As vertebral osteomyelitis progresses and can lead to local tissue destruction and sepsis, it is important to closely follow patients at risk with repeat evaluation and testing within 2 weeks of initial presentation.

The mainstay of treatment for vertebral osteomyelitis is antibiotics. In any individual with vertebral osteomyelitis who is not septic and who is neurologically intact, it is recommended to delay antibiotic treatment until a causative pathogen has been found. The simplest way to identify the culprit is by obtaining blood cultures, but these often do not yield an organism, even with specific culture techniques as might be clinically appropriate (e.g. fungal blood cultures in a patient with immunocompromise and a chronic peripherally inserted central catheter (PICC)). If blood cultures remain negative, or if a polymicrobial infection is suspected, the next step is to obtain a tissue sample through biopsy, either percutaneously with CT guidance or via open biopsy in the operating room. Aside from open biopsy, other clear indications for surgery include progressive neurologic compromise and gross spinal instability. Unfortunately, there are little definitive data to guide decision-making around prescribing antibiotics, pursuing biopsy, and considering surgery. Given the high stakes involved, in any patient with identified or highly suspected vertebral osteomyelitis, it is essential to urgently involve both an infectious disease physician and a spine surgeon (orthopedic or neurosurgical). Depending on the circumstances, the best way to involve these specialists may be a phone call, a secure message, urgent referral to their clinic, or consultation in the emergency department.

Outcomes vary depending in part on baseline medical and sociodemographic factors. The mortality rate of vertebral osteomyelitis is approximately 6% and nearly one-third of patients have persistent complications, most commonly pain or neurologic deficit. As described in a recent study of inpatient hospitalizations in the United States, an increased rate of mortality during the initial hospitalization was associated with age greater than 80 years, male sex, and medical comorbidities including congestive heart failure, cerebrovascular disease, liver disease, and kidney disease. Extended length of stay in the hospital (and higher costs) was associated with age greater than 80 years, Hispanic ethnicity, Black race, and medical comorbidities.

For the patient in this case, the 45-year-old man on a TNF-alpha inhibitor who has new onset LBP and persistent fatigue following a recent bacterial pneumonia, we started with vital signs and a neuromusculoskeletal physical exam, which was unremarkable. We explained to the patient that we were concerned about possible infection, and we ordered ESR, CRP, and plain X-rays of the lumbar spine, which were obtained immediately. Both lab tests came back elevated. An emergent MRI of the lumbar spine with and without IV contrast was obtained, showing abnormalities at L2/L3 consistent with an infection, including findings in the disc and adjacent bone and psoas abscesses (see Figures 15.1 and 15.2).

At this point, we contacted the hospital's on-call infectious disease physician and arranged for direct hospital admission for further workup and management. Blood cultures were drawn, and IV antibiotics were initiated based on the known organism that had caused his pneumonia, subsequently confirmed from the blood cultures. Orthopedic spine surgery was also consulted, and they recommended nonsurgical care with follow-up in their clinic in 3–4 weeks. He was discharged from the hospital within a few days with an anticipated course of antibiotics for 6–8 weeks under the care of his infectious disease specialist.

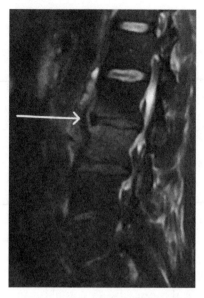

FIGURE 15.1. MRI image, T2 sequence, sagittal view. There is brightness in the anterior inferior endplate of the L2 vertebra and throughout the vertebral body of L3 with an associated area of brightness anteriorly to the L2/L3 intervertebral disc (white arrow).

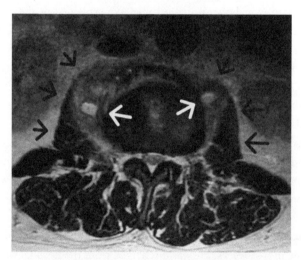

FIGURE 15.2. MRI image of the same individual in Figure 15.1, T2 sequence, axial view, at the level of the L2/L3 disc. Within the right and left psoas muscles (muscle borders denoted by black arrows), there is an irregularly defined region of relative brightness emanating from the disc. This region enhances on post-contrast imaging (not shown), corroborating a diagnostic impression of phlegmon. Bilaterally within the phlegmon there are well demarcated fluid collections consistent with intramuscular abscesses (white arrows).

1. Concerning historical features for the presence of vertebral osteomyelitis include intravenous drug use, diabetes mellitus, immune compromise, and recent bacterial infection.
2. Patients with vertebral osteomyelitis usually present with local pain without neurological deficits, and many patients are afebrile.
3. Erythrocyte sedimentation rate (ESR) and C-reactive protein (CRP) have excellent sensitivity for vertebral osteomyelitis so are a good pair of screening tests.
4. The preferred diagnostic imaging modality for suspected vertebral osteomyelitis is magnetic resonance imaging (MRI) with intravenous gadolinium contrast.
5. In a patient with vertebral osteomyelitis who is non-septic and who is neurologically intact, it is recommended to delay initiation of antibiotics until after blood cultures have been drawn.

Further reading
1. Berbari EF, Kanj SS, Kowalski TJ, et al. 2015 Infectious Disease Society of America (IDSA) clinical practice guidelines for the diagnosis and treatment of native vertebral osteomyelitis in adult. Clin Infect Dis. 2013;61:e26–e46. doi: 10.1093/cid/civ482.
2. Issa K, Diebo B, Faloon M, et al. The epidemiology of vertebral osteomyelitis in the United States from 1998 to 2013. Clin Spine Surg. 2018 Mar;31(2):e102–e108. doi: 10.1097/BSD.0000000000000597.
3. Maamari J, Tande AJ, Diehn F, Tai DBG, Berbari EF. Diagnosis of vertebral osteomyelitis. J Bone Joint Infect. 2022;7:23–32. doi: 10.5194/jbji-7-23-2022.
4. Mylona E, Samarkos M, Kakalou E, Fanourgiakis P, Skoutelis A. Pyogenic vertebral osteomyelitis: a systematic review of clinical characteristics. Semin Arthrit Rheum. 2009;39:10–17. doi: 10.1016/j.semarthrit.2008.03.002.
5. Zimmerli W. "Osteomyelitis." In *Harrison's Principles of Internal Medicine*, edited by J Loscalzo, A Fauci, D Kasper, S Hauser, D Longo, JL Jameson. McGraw Hill; 2022. Accessed May 21, 2023. https://accessmedicine.mhmedical.com/content.aspx?bookid=3095&sectionid=265415427.

16 "I'm Really Scared.": Acute Back and Leg Pain with Incontinence

Charles Reitman

Your nurse just informed you about an urgent call from a patient with acute back pain and incontinence. You call the patient, and they report the acute onset of severe low back pain with loss of bladder control shortly after. This has never happened before. The pain is accompanied by paresthesia into both legs. The patient can walk but feels a bit unsteady. The pain started after a brief coughing spell just a few hours ago. They note no significant history of back pain in the past and no ongoing or acute medical problems. The patient is concerned and wants to know what you recommend.

What do you do now?

This patient presents with a clinical picture consistent with cauda equina syndrome (CES). This is a clinical diagnosis that represents dysfunction of the nervous system at the level of the cauda equina. Symptoms include bowel and bladder dysfunction, sensory changes (particularly in the perineum but can include the lower extremities), and possible loss of distal motor function in the lower extremities. Patients often report pain in the back, buttocks, and/or lower extremities, but not always, and the hallmark features are the signs and symptoms related to neurological deterioration.

Anatomically, the spinal cord is an extension of the brain. The spinal cord ends at the conus medullaris which is a collection of the cell bodies of the lumbar and sacral motor nerve roots. The conus begins in the lower thoracic spine and usually terminates around the level of the L1/L2 disc space, although this can be variable. The cauda equina (Latin for "horse's tail") is then the collection of the lumbar and sacral nerve roots that travel distally from the conus in the thecal sac and exit at their respective levels in the lumbar and sacral spines. While chronic CES can have more variable etiologies, acute or subacute onset CES is almost always due to a relatively abrupt compression of the thecal sac, generally from conditions including but not limited to disc herniation, epidural hematoma, tumor, or infection.

While the typical radiographic features involve severe thecal sac compression, CES is not a radiographic diagnosis, and regardless of the severity of the radiographic stenosis, CES does not exist in the absence of clinical symptoms and signs. As a result of the compression on the thecal sac, prominent symptoms of sacral root compression occur, including bowel and bladder dysfunction along with perineal numbness. The lumbar symptoms are more variable and can include pain, weakness, or sensory changes in the lower extremities.

This patient needs an immediate evaluation. It is acceptable for this initial evaluation to occur in an outpatient office setting if it can be arranged the same day; but, if not, this patient should be evaluated in the emergency room. Advantages to office evaluation are that it is usually more expeditious than navigating through the emergency room and that you can clarify the details and the accuracy of the history to prompt further emergent assessment. An advantage to the emergency room is that the patient is already in the hospital if they need further advanced imaging and eventual admission for urgent surgery.

A thorough neurological exam should be conducted. Consistent with their subjective complaints, the hallmark findings include sensory loss in the perineal region and, less consistently, in the lower extremities, as well as motor loss. Motor loss includes diminished rectal tone but can also variably include decreased strength in the lower extremities. Reflexes are also variably affected and may be normal or depressed. CES does not result in upper motor neuron findings. Therefore, the presence of findings such as hyperreflexia, clonus, or upgoing toes with Babinski test suggest a lesion at the spinal cord level or higher. Straight leg raising may result in leg pain, but, again, this is variable and not differentiating in any way. Trunk range-of-motion can also be variably affected and is not critical to making the diagnosis.

It is never wrong to obtain X-rays of the lumbar spine in patients presenting with neurological symptoms consistent with a lumbar spine origin. However, in the presence of significant neurological changes, advanced imaging is most appropriate as a first line study. Magnetic resonance imaging (MRI) without contrast is the gold standard imaging study. If there is high suspicion of tumor or infection, addition of intravenous contrast is appropriate. If there is a problem getting a contrast study quickly, speed is more important, and the non-contrast study will be adequate. If the patient cannot have an MRI, myelogram and post myelogram computed tomography (CT) would be the next most preferred study. If there are contraindications to both MRI and administration of myelographic contrast dye, then a plain CT scan will suffice. CT scans are usually readily accessible, quick, and accommodate patients of almost any weight. Without myelographic contrast dye, however, they lack detail of the spinal canal and nerve roots, and it may be more difficult to reliably assess compromise of the cauda equina. Electrodiagnostic studies have no role as a first line test for diagnosis of this condition. While CES is a clinical diagnosis, imaging is absolutely necessary to confirm the diagnosis and direct decision-making. Laboratory data are not necessary to make the diagnosis but may be helpful in the setting of possible infection or cancer.

To confirm CES, you are looking for alignment of all data, including symptoms, decreased perianal sensation, bladder and/or bowel dysfunction, possible neurological decline in lower extremity function, and imaging findings. True diminished perianal sensation and decreased or absent rectal tone and sphincter contraction are the main features. Although urinary incontinence can have a variety of etiologies, suspicion for CES should be high if accompanied by exam findings of decreased perianal sensation or decreased rectal tone. With a clinical picture consistent with CES, imaging can confirm the diagnosis. Canal stenosis should be present and, in general CES, occurs more frequently from acute canal stenosis than from degenerative changes that gradually affect the spinal canal over time. Most often the acute stenosis seen on imaging would be caused by an acute disc herniation, epidural hematoma, epidural abscess, or expansion of a tumor (see Figure 16.1).

Patients that present with a deteriorating neurological exam have an underlying problem that is time-sensitive. To that end, evaluation should proceed expeditiously, and consulting the appropriate specialists early is essential, in this case an orthopedic surgeon or neurosurgeon. There is an old saying in these progressive neurologic conditions that "time is neurons," so engaging specialists early can and does change the final outcome. If patients present with this declining neurological picture in the absence of spinal stenosis, alternative neurological processes, such as acute inflammatory

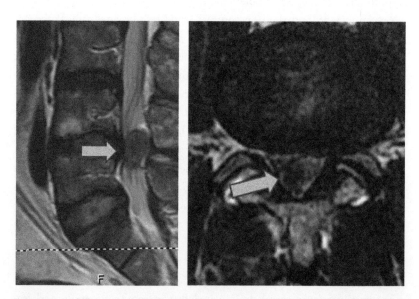

FIGURE 16.1. MRI images showing a large disc herniation at L4/L5 (arrows). Mid-sagittal (A) and axial image at the L4/L5 level (B). The disc herniation occupies essentially the entire spinal canal.

demyelinating polyradiculoneuropathy (AIDP, also Guillain-Barre Syndrome), should be considered, and a neurologist should be consulted.

If a patient has symptoms and physical examination findings consistent with CES and severe spinal stenosis on imaging findings, this is a surgical emergency. Although surgery should be performed as quickly as possible, surgery can be appropriately delayed for a short period of time for specific reasons. There are data that suggest that long-term outcomes may be similar with surgical intervention up to 2 days following onset of symptoms. However, unless there is an important reason to wait, the earlier the intervention, the better. As soon as you are aware of a progressive neurological deficit, the patient's diet should be held as should anticoagulant medications. Medical comorbidities should be identified and optimized to reduce risk of surgical complications or worse outcomes following surgery.

Corticosteroids are often used in the presence of acute neurological deterioration. In the case of acute CES, there are no data for or against the use of steroids. Early surgical intervention is the priority. In the absence of any data, use of oral Corticosteroids is reasonable if there are no contraindications otherwise. In general, medication to protect the gastrointestinal system should be given in combination if corticosteroids are used.

Surgery will include a decompression of the thecal sac. Additional stabilization of the spine may be necessary depending on the underlying disease. Outcomes are usually favorable but are directly related to speed of intervention and the severity of symptoms and signs at the time of surgery. With early intervention, you can usually expect improvement in neurological function, although there may be incomplete recovery. Bowel, bladder, and sexual function (i.e. sacral nerve functions) are the least resilient, typically take the longest to recover, and are most likely to exhibit permanent impairment.

KEY POINTS

1. Acute CES is a clinical diagnosis that includes progressive loss of neurological function of the lumbosacral nerves resulting in perineal numbness, incontinence of bladder and/or bowel, and

variable loss of lower limb strength, sensation, and function. It may or may not be associated with significant pain.

2. Although there are other medical conditions that can mimic CES, mechanical compression of the lumbar thecal sac is the most common cause, and final diagnosis is based on the clinical exam and supportive imaging.

3. MRI is the imaging study of choice to confirm compression of the cauda equina. CT myelogram or a CT scan, in that order, can be considered if the preferential tests are contraindicated.

4. Progressive loss of neurological function is an emergency, and evaluation and treatment should proceed expeditiously without delay.

5. As a first responder, hold diet and anticoagulation medications until a definitive treatment plan is established as emergency surgery is likely needed. Evaluate and optimize any other medical conditions to the best of your ability in anticipation of possible emergency surgical intervention.

Further reading
1. Kuris E, McDonald C, Palumbo M, Daniels A. Evaluation and management of cauda equina syndrome. Am J Med. 2021;134(12):1483–1489.
2. Long B, Koyfman A, Gottlieb M. Evaluation and management of cauda equina syndrome in the emergency department. Am J Emerg Med. 2020;38:143–148.
3. Spector L, Madigan L, Rhyne A, Darden B, Kim D. Cauda equina syndrome. J Am Acad Ortho Surg. 2008;16:471–479.
4. Srikandarajah N, Wilby M, Clark S, Noble A. Williamson P, Marson T. Outcomes reported after surgery for cauda equina syndrome. A systematic literature review. Spine. 2018;43:E1005–1013.
5. Todd N. Guidelines for cauda equina syndrome. Red flags and white flags. Systematic review and implications for triage. Br J Neurosurg. 2017;31:336–339.

17 "I Just Keep Getting Worse.": Long-Standing Depression and Progressive Low Back Pain

Laura M. Tuck, Moriah J. Brier, Erica Ho, Derek R. Anderson, Rhonda M. Williams, Christopher J. Standaert, Aaron P. Turner

A 54-year-old presents with ongoing low back pain for the past year. They "can't do anything" because of the pain. It increases with any activity. There is no leg pain or neurologic loss. The patient has a history of depression since adolescence. They have tried numerous medications over time and currently take a serotonin and norepinephrine reuptake inhibitor (SNRI). Despite this, the depression screen obtained by your office indicates moderate to severe depression and elevated anxiety. They live alone, work as a shipping clerk, and are evasive about questions on alcohol use. There is no history of trauma, cancer, or infection. The patient notes "physical therapy never helps" and that they do not exercise regularly.

Chiropractic in the past was unhelpful. On physical exam, mood and affect are blunted, neurologic exam is normal, and any flexion of the lumbar spine is accompanied by pain. X-rays from 8 months ago show loss of disc height at L4/L5 and L5/S1 with normal alignment.

What do you do now?

The comorbid presentation of chronic low back pain (LBP) and depression is common. Many estimates suggest over half of patients with chronic pain also have major depression. Chronic pain can lead to or exacerbate low mood through decreased engagement in valued activity, loss of function in work, family, and social life, and poor sleep.[1] Depression, in turn, can contribute to the maintenance of chronic pain through social withdrawal, negative thinking, and reduced activity. In this case, anxiety is also elevated, which is a common comorbidity with both chronic pain and depression. Mutually reinforcing neurobiological pathways associated with all three of these conditions contribute to aggravation and maintenance of symptom severity.

Regardless of "which comes first," individuals with comorbid mental health concerns and chronic pain, particularly when either or both conditions are long-standing, are among the most complex patients to treat. Effective treatment entails a multifaceted approach focused on improving function, insight into the interrelationship between pain and mental health issues, self-efficacy in sustained lifestyle changes, and establishing clear functional goals. This requires patient receptiveness and engagement in the philosophy of care and should be viewed as a collaborative process between patients and providers. Patients who feel invalidated by the health care system are less likely to engage in adaptive health behaviors and are at an increased risk for perpetuating the "medical merry go round" of unnecessary testing and interventions.

Neither pain nor depression can be treated in isolation. Primary care providers will need to address both simultaneously even if a psychologist or other mental health provider collaborates in care. Similarly, any involved mental health providers will need to address depression and anxiety in the specific context of having comorbid chronic pain. Only by appreciating these conditions as linked can both be effectively understood and managed. The complexities of comorbid depression and chronic pain are often most effectively addressed through a holistic and individually tailored biopsychosocial approach. This typically begins with an interview or conversation assessing function and biological, psychological, and social/contextual factors, such as an injury history, medical comorbidities, life stressors, mental health symptoms, social support, and personal goals. Thoughtful assessment can foster rapport and promote patient engagement, illuminate readiness for a collaborative/self-management approach, and elicit diagnostic concerns, treatment preferences, pain beliefs, and functional goals.

During assessment, empathically educate the patient that pain is not just a biological experience but is also influenced by psychological and social factors. Education can be both general and specific to their concerns. For example, in this case, it may involve reassuring the patient about the absence of "red flags" on imaging. Note that loss of disc height on imaging is common in people with and without pain, is benign, and is not predictive of worsening pain. Discuss the differences between acute and chronic pain and inform the patient that the central goal of treatment will focus on improved function and quality of life and not on pain elimination. Reassure the patient that despite not being able to eliminate pain, their team will continue to monitor and provide ongoing care. Set the stage for using active (rather than passive) pain management strategies, which support the patient's ability to develop confidence and skills in managing pain independently. Active treatments include self-management skills, such as a home exercise program and coping skills, and are correlated with long-term functional gains.

Take the time perhaps over multiple meetings to express compassion and understand the subjective experience of the patient, including losses and challenges. Ask open-ended questions such as, "What do you miss doing?" and "How has chronic pain affected your identity?" Additional assessment considerations that highlight the overlap within domains of the biopsychosocial model as possible maintaining factors of the pain and depression cycles include the role of medical comorbidities such as long-standing or life-threatening illness, sleep disorders, endocrine dysfunction, cognitive changes and suboptimal medications.

An effective patient-provider relationship requires trust and respect, which cannot exist without sensitivity and appreciation of the importance of diversity. Throughout your discussion with the patient, acknowledge individual and systemic factors that may contribute to their experiences, in both positive and negative ways. For instance, if someone belongs to a marginalized group and/or has suffered trauma or abuse, it is likely they have experienced discrimination, confusion, disappointment, or even harm within the health care system. Examine and critically reflect on how your own identity characteristics may impact: 1) the patient's experience and their level of comfort in working with you (and your comfort in working with them); and 2) your perceptions of their behaviors. Ask questions that convey a sense of openness and humility. For example, consider asking whether the patient knows anyone who has gone through similar issues before, and about any personal, familial, or cultural beliefs surrounding health, sickness, and pain. Ask about strengths or protective attributes the patient draws from their unique identity characteristics. Invite the patient to share with you and the health care team what they feel is most important for you to understand about them.

Motivational interviewing (MI) is recommended to improve engagement in active treatment.[2] MI is a communication technique used to elicit behavior change through exploration of values-based decision-making that is designed to minimize resistance and increase commitment. Ask questions like "We've discussed a lot of strategies today. Which one would you be willing to try?" Highlight the consequences of inaction by inquiring "What is the cost of NOT doing that?" Use MI when forming initial treatment goals followed by routine check-ins on treatment gains and barriers. Using MI techniques in conversations with the patient can be a helpful clinical approach and may aid in focusing the patient on active approaches to care, enhancing self-efficacy, and establishing meaningful goals.

Common to both chronic pain and depression is a style of thinking known as catastrophizing, in which patients habitually "think the worst" about their experience. Pain catastrophizing refers to thoughts that include rumination about pain, magnifying the intensity of pain, and/or feeling a sense of helplessness about pain. These negative thoughts can in turn lead to kinesiophobia, or fear of movement, and result in higher levels of pain and disability through worsening mood and deactivation—in other words, a pattern of fear and avoidance. Mental health providers treating depression and chronic pain target catastrophizing and avoidance directly by using empirically supported approaches, described below. Primary care providers also play a key role in countering catastrophizing thoughts and bolstering self-efficacy by emphasizing that patients can develop skills to better manage their pain and that hurt does not equal harm when engaging in activity. When the relationship between pain and mental health is recognized, treatment is more effective.

For this individual, thorough assessment of psychological factors is key. Depression is an important focus of care given its severity, long duration, pre-pain onset, and prominent role in deactivation maintaining the chronic pain cycle. Elevated levels of anxiety are also notable, as they may play a role in avoiding activity and engagement in treatment. Assessment of suicidal risk is critical because depression and chronic pain are known risk factors for self-harm. Evidence suggests that suicide rates are twice as high among those with chronic pain. A contributing factor to higher suicide rates may be problematic alcohol use, which can contribute to depression and pain and reduce the effectiveness of pharmacologic and behavioral treatments. Assess alcohol use with a brief screening measure such as the Alcohol Use Disorders Identification Test (AUDIT-C) with established clinical cutoffs.

This patient is experiencing high levels of pain, depression, possible alcohol misuse, and declines in function and health. They would likely benefit from working with a behavioral health provider, such as a clinical psychologist or clinical social worker, to address these issues collectively with an emphasis on depressive symptoms. There are several effective pain-focused psychotherapies to address chronic pain, depression, and anxiety which may include cognitive behavioral therapy for chronic pain, acceptance and commitment therapy for chronic pain, mindfulness meditation and hypnosis.[3–6] In cases of long-standing moderate to severe depression, such as with this patient, engagement with mental health for focused depression treatment may also be indicated.

Increased physical activity is a critical area of intervention for patients with chronic pain and depression and counters avoidance from both etiologies. Reassure the patient that increasing physical activity will not cause harm. Referral to physical therapy can help the patient gain self-efficacy through learning time-based pacing for both exercise and general activity. Physical activity should be discussed with the patient in a collaborative fashion, as simply providing information and recommendations is typically insufficient to create lasting behavior change. As there is no "perfect" exercise, starting with exercise patients enjoy and can access is more likely to be successful. As reported by this patient, many patients are dissatisfied with PT due to having unrealistic expectations for significant pain reduction. Provide education that the goal of PT is functional gains. For this patient,

PT should focus on pain neuroeducation, reducing kinesiophobia, pacing, and goal-directed exercise. In addition to promoting function, physical activity has a demonstrated positive impact on depression.

In terms of medications, opioids are not recommended for this patient due to safety concerns, poor evidence of long-term efficacy, and risk of opioid induced hyperalgesia. Long-term opioid use can also increase the risk of depression and maintain symptoms. Muscle relaxants lose effectiveness over time and should be used sparingly. This patient is already taking a SNRI, which can address pain and mood while reducing polypharmacy. Ensure this patient's dose is at a therapeutic level. Higher doses improve mood, but not necessarily pain. If depression or anxiety are inadequately treated with current medication, consider referral to a psychiatrist. Be mindful of prescribing medications that may reduce activity due to sedating effects, disrupt sleep, or increase risk for suicide. The effectiveness of antidepressants, psychotherapy, and exercise for depression is increased when used in combination.

Withdrawal from activities and relationships maintains both chronic pain and depression. Engagement in meaningful activity can protect against functional impairment stemming from either. Affirm this patient's efforts to maintain productivity at their job. Social support is associated with myriad health benefits. It is notable that this patient lives alone. Explore the patient's emotional, companionship, informational, and financial supports and how these relationships may bolster functioning or maintain the pain cycle. If social support is limited, explore possible ways the patient might cultivate a richer social support network and engagement in meaningful activity.

In summary, as this patient has no medical "red flags," such as neurologic or musculoskeletal concerns, there is likely very little, if any, role for interventional pain approaches or surgery. The preferred approach is supporting self-management through skills development and lifestyle modification. These can be addressed via educating the patient about the interrelationship between pain and depression, exploring psychosocial barriers and strengths to support functional gains, engaging them in a goal-directed approach to activity, and focusing on improvement of function and quality of life. Additional support via stand alone or integrated mental health (where available) is indicated.

1. Assess biological, psychological, and social factors contributing to this patient's pain experience and provide education about the interrelationship between pain and depression.
2. Focus treatment on improving function and not on pain elimination.
3. Emphasize active treatments over passive ones. Support a path toward self-management.
4. Reassure the patient that movement is safe and encourage paced reactivation.
5. Prioritize treatment of the patient's underlying depression.

Further reading

1. Von Korff M, Simon G. The relationship between pain and depression. Br J Psych. 1996;168:101–108.
2. Miller W, Rollnick S. *Motivational Interviewing*, 3rd ed. New York, NY: Guilford Press, 2013.
3. Burch V, Penman D. *You Are Not Your Pain: Using Mindfulness to Relieve Pain, Reduce Stress, and Restore Well-Being—an Eight-Week Program*. New York, NY: Macmillan, 2015.
4. Dahl J, Luciano C, Wilson K. *Acceptance and Commitment Therapy for Chronic Pain*. Reno, NY: New Harbinger Publications, 2005.
5. Jensen, M. *Hypnosis for Chronic Pain Management*. New York, NY: Oxford University Press, 2011.
6. Otis, J. *Managing Chronic Pain: A Cognitive-Behavioral Therapy Approach*. New York, NY: Oxford University Press, 2007.

18 "I Know I Have Fibromyalgia, but My Back Hurts.": Back Pain and Fibromyalgia

Christopher J. Standaert, Isaiah Levy

A 46-year-old female with a history of widespread pain requests help for her low back. She notes a long history of pain in her neck, shoulders, low back, hip, and several other joints, along with fatigue and poor sleep. After a thorough laboratory study for possible rheumatologic conditions 10 years ago, she was diagnosed with fibromyalgia. She has taken over the counter analgesics and "muscle relaxers" in the past without tremendous benefit. She has never found physical therapy helpful, and she struggles with limited activity tolerance, fatigue, and pain. She maintains her job as a freelance writer and walks for exercise when not limited by pain or fatigue, which is maybe once per week. Her low back has been painful for the past few months. There was no trauma, she has not been ill, has no history of cancer, and her weight is stable. She has some radiation of pain to the left posterior hip at times but mostly lower back pain with no numbness or weakness or other neurologic change.

What do you do now?

ow back pain (LBP) and fibromyalgia coexist in many patients, and the majority of those with fibromyalgia experience LBP. The frequencies of depression, anxiety, PTSD, and trauma are elevated in the populations of individuals with fibromyalgia and with chronic LBP compared to those without chronic pain. Additionally, psychological factors including pain catastrophization and kinesiophobia are causally implicated in the pain-related disability for those with either chronic LBP or fibromyalgia. Despite this overlap, however, those with fibromyalgia are also prone to the same spinal issues as the rest of the population, such as disc herniations, spondylolisthesis, and others. From a diagnostic perspective, it is critical that providers do not routinely assume all pain in those with fibromyalgia is solely related to that disorder. It is equally important to be aware of the need to approach treatment differently in someone with a history of fibromyalgia or other chronic pain disorders than in those who do not have the same experience of pain.

Fibromyalgia is characterized by widespread/multifocal pain, frequently associated with other somatic symptoms like sleep disturbance, fatigue, and cognitive dysfunction. It is increasingly considered a disorder of central sensitization with disturbances of pain processing and regulation. The estimated prevalence in the general population is about 2% with a roughly 2:1 female to male predominance. Population estimates are challenged by the lack of a clear, objective gold standard for diagnosis, however.

There have been numerous diagnostic criteria proposed across multiple professional medical associations and countries since 1990. The criteria have progressed from an initial focus on tenderness to palpation to self-reported pain and other symptoms. Despite this evolution, the diagnostic criteria have remained somewhat subjective and are inconsistently applied across the health care system. Using the 2011 American College of Rheumatology criteria for the diagnosis of fibromyalgia, a large US population survey found that almost 75% of those reporting a diagnosis of fibromyalgia did not meet diagnostic criteria for the disorder. A survey of practicing physicians found a very poor overall understanding of published diagnostic criteria. About 50% of the physicians in this survey did not use any criteria whatsoever to make the diagnosis but simply relied on their overall clinical impression. Unfortunately, the central role of expert opinion in diagnosis contributes to uncertainty, inconsistency, skepticism, and bias, all of which can be perceived by both patients and providers.

Bias is reflected in clinical practice. The degree to which there is a female predominance for the diagnosis is often overestimated, potentially leading to women being falsely diagnosed with fibromyalgia and men being underdiagnosed. In one study, 90% of patients referred to a specialty clinic for possible fibromyalgia were women, a gross distortion of the actual predominance of 2:1 in women compared to men. In the United States, ethnic minorities diagnosed with fibromyalgia tend to have worse levels of pain, depression, and sleep disturbance than those who are White. Women with a low educational or socioeconomic status are also referred for multimodal pain treatment at lower rates than those of high educational attainment or income.

From a therapeutic standpoint, fibromyalgia, like LBP, is best approached as a biopsychosocial disorder. It is generally recommended that treatment should focus on improving quality of life and function while managing symptoms, more so than "curing" the disorder. This includes addressing exercise, sleep, stress, diet, and pacing using a multimodal approach. Managing concurrent issues such as major depression, anxiety, post-traumatic stress disorder (PTSD), and fear avoidance—all common in those with chronic pain—is also an important component of care. Tricyclic antidepressants and pregabalin have been shown to be helpful in addressing pain and sleep in those with fibromyalgia, and duloxetine may help in treating pain and depression. These medications benefit a minority of patients, however, and may be associated with side effects. Cognitive behavioral therapy can offer benefit. As in chronic LBP, overly "medicalizing" the diagnosis of fibromyalgia, in this case as strictly an issue of neural hypersensitivity, can lead to the neglect of important psychological and social contributors to both pain and disability.

In considering the patient presented here, she is 46 years old with an existing diagnosis of fibromyalgia. The details used to make that diagnosis are not clear, so there may be an issue with its validity. However, the patient has had multifocal chronic pain and what she legitimately understands to be fibromyalgia for 10 years or so. Whether one wishes to revisit the diagnosis or not, which may be both unhelpful and unnecessary for her current presentation, this patient likely has a component of central sensitization that influences her pain experience and is at relatively high risk of having a coexistent mental health disorder like major depression or PTSD. Although she tries to stay active and continues to work, she also has limited activity tolerance and is probably substantially deconditioned. She has been through relatively ineffective treatment for pain in the past, including physical therapy and analgesics. This may influence her receptiveness to these approaches being used to help her LBP. The degree to which she believes that her current low back issues can improve, her level of fear avoidance or illness conviction, and ongoing psychosocial drivers of pain and disability are also issues that need to be explored, given her long-standing history of persistent pain.

Although limited, existing data indicate that patients with fibromyalgia often have relatively negative experiences with the health care system, ranging from ineffective care to uncertainty about the diagnosis, disregard, and lack of providers perceived as having sufficient knowledge about the diagnosis. Many patients are subsequently afraid to pursue medical care for fibromyalgia because of these issues. In order to help this patient with her LBP, she will need to feel that her story is heard, that her concerns are addressed, and that her pain is assessed as a legitimate problem and not swept into her experience with fibromyalgia.

In thinking about her spine, we have to consider how to approach persistent subacute to chronic LBP as an initial presentation. Given her age, she may be at risk for a variety of spine-related processes. Disc herniations are relatively common in the mid-40s. Although on the younger end for those with extensive age-associated degenerative process, conditions including a degenerative spondylolisthesis, degenerative scoliosis, or hip osteoarthritis need to be considered. She does have pain into her left gluteal area, which may either be referred from her L4/L5 or L5/S1 spinal segments (any structure from these levels can refer pain to the posterior gluteal area) or from a structure in the pelvis or posterior hip. Although slightly older than those typically presenting with the acute onset of a spondyloarthropathy, this could be a consideration. Given that she has more LBP than gluteal/pelvic pain, an isolated pelvic process like sacroiliitis, a sacral fracture, or gluteal muscle strain all seem less likely. She has no history of spinal trauma, cancer, or other "red flag" type issues.

Physical examination should include an evaluation of her spine for possible scoliosis or other postural abnormalities, palpation for focal tenderness (although this has to be interpreted with caution, given her history), observation of her gait, examination of the range of motion of her spine and her hips, and a neurological examination of the lower extremities. As she has had a distinct increase in her LBP for several months, further diagnostic evaluation with plain radiographs is appropriate. Standing radiographs to include antero-posterior and lateral flexion/extension views should be obtained if radiographs are pursued. Given the absence of any urgent neurological or red flag issues, there is no indication for advanced imaging such as magnetic resonance imaging (MRI) at this point. Unless a clear medical or rheumatologic concern is identified in the history and examination, there is also no indication for laboratory studies.

In this case, she adds that her symptoms are worse with standing than sitting or lying down and came on gradually. She has become increasingly more sedentary with mild weight gain over the last few months. Her home and work situations are stable and secure, but her mood has declined as her pain has increased. She is neurologically intact, hip range of motion is normal, her lumbar region is diffusely tender to palpation, and she may have an underlying curve/scoliosis noted. She is a bit hesitant to bend either forward or backwards in standing. Her radiographs show a mild convex left lumbar scoliosis of 15 degrees with a slight degenerative spondylolisthesis of 3 mm at L4/L5 without instability on flexion/extension views and mild multilevel degenerative change.

Although potentially notable, these radiologic findings are frequently seen in individuals without LBP (see chapter 4 for a discussion of radiographic findings, chapter 9 for a discussion of degenerative spondylolisthesis, and chapter 10 for a discussion of scoliosis). Given her history, it is difficult to specifically ascribe her pain to any of these findings, and care should be taken to explain them as issues that are seen in many women her age without LBP. However, her pain could be related to these issues, and all of them are amenable to the rehabilitation approach described below. Were her symptoms to subsequently involve leg pain or neurological concerns, postural changes, or worsening pain over the next 6–12 months, repeat radiographs and an MRI may be indicated. Degenerative spondylolisthesis and degenerative scoliosis can progress and become more symptomatic over time.

At the moment, care should focus on conservative measures intended to improve her engagement in exercise, sleep, and diet. Fear and depressed mood should be addressed concurrently. These issues overlap with the more chronic concerns of her fibromyalgia diagnosis, but she has had a relatively acute functional decline that needs to be addressed. NSAIDs can be reintroduced as an option for her more acute back symptoms, distinguishing those from her widespread pain. Duloxetine could be a useful medication given the potential for benefit for her LBP, fibromyalgia, and depression. A physical therapy referral is appropriate. This has to focus on the gradual introduction of low impact cardiovascular exercise, gentle range of motion, and basic strengthening exercises for her trunk. Aquatic therapy would be an excellent setting for initial physical therapy. A psychology referral to address fear, pacing, and goal setting may be helpful.

She needs to understand the importance of consistent activity in both restoration of function and maintenance of her spine and long-term health. She will need to start an exercise program at a level that does not worsen her pain and can be maintained at least three times per week. This may be only a short walk or 5–10 minutes on a stationary bike, for example, but this can then be gradually increased over time. If sleep hygiene has not previously been optimized as part of addressing her fibromyalgia, this should be explored. Nutritional support to optimize her diet would also be appropriate. As she has likely found much of this unhelpful for her widespread symptoms in the past, it is worth discussing that these steps are important for her spine and that she may find benefit for her spine that is distinct from her prior experience. If the spondylolisthesis or scoliosis plays a role in her current pain, exercise and weight optimization would be primary long-term approaches to managing both of these. There is no indication for a spinal injection or surgery currently. Opiates should be avoided. In order to provide ongoing support, assess the response to or need for medications, and allow for additional steps in care, she should return for follow-up relatively frequently as she goes through physical therapy.

KEY POINTS

1. Fibromyalgia is characterized by widespread pain, associated somatic symptoms, and likely central sensitization of pain pathways.

2. The diagnosis of fibromyalgia is complicated by multiple criteria and provider reliance on expert or personal opinion.
3. New spine or other musculoskeletal complaints in those with fibromyalgia need to be evaluated independently and not routinely ascribed to fibromyalgia.
4. Treatment of LBP in those with fibromyalgia has to incorporate an understanding and validation of the patient's experience with both pain and the health care system.
5. Physical limitations, behavioral health comorbidities, and belief structures may influence treatment recommendations and engagement in care in those with LBP and fibromyalgia.

Further reading
1. Hackshaw K. Assessing our approach to diagnosing fibromyalgia. Expert Rev Mol Diagn. 2020;20(12):1171–1181. doi:10.1080/14737159.2020.1858054.
2. Hasselroth R, Björling G, Faag C, Bose CN. "Can someone as young as you really feel that much pain?"—a survey on how people with fibromyalgia experience healthcare in Sweden. SAGE Open Nurs. 2021 Jun 24;7:23779608211026145. doi: 10.1177/23779608211026145.
3. Kumbhare D, Ahmed S, Sander T, et al. A survey of physicians' knowledge and adherence to the diagnostic criteria for fibromyalgia. Pain Med. 2018;19(6):1254–1264.
4. Walitt B, Katz RS, Bergman MJ, Wolfe F. Three-quarters of persons in the US population reporting a clinical diagnosis of fibromyalgia do not satisfy fibromyalgia criteria: the 2012 National Health Interview Survey. PLoS One. 2016 Jun 9;11(6):e0157235. doi: 10.1371/journal.pone.0157235.
5. Wolfe F, Clauw DJ, Fitzcharles MA, et al. 2016 Revisions to the 2010/2011 fibromyalgia diagnostic criteria. Semin Arthritis Rheum. 2016 Dec;46(3):319–329. doi: 10.1016/j.semarthrit.2016.08.012. Epub 2016 Aug 30.

19 "I Was Rear-Ended Last Week, and My Back Is Killing Me.": Pain after a Motor Vehicle Accident

Benjamin D. Holmes, Steven J. Atlas,

Eric J. Roseen

An otherwise healthy 31-year-old male presents with acute low back pain. He notes he was injured in a motor vehicle collision 1 week ago. He was stopped at a red light when he was hit from behind. He thought he was okay at the scene, although he thinks he "was in a state of shock." He was ambulatory after the collision. A friend drove him home as his car "was totaled." He shows you pictures of his damaged car that are on his cell phone. He notes he woke up the following day stiff all over and gradually developed pain across his low back over the next day or two. He has largely been in bed or on the couch the last 5 days and has not gone to work. He states, "My back is killing me." He has no leg symptoms, neurologic complaints, or prior back issues, and he has not pursued other medical care since the accident. He is taking over the counter nonsteroidal anti-inflammatory medications at doses higher than standardly prescribed. His gait and movements are guarded.

Low back pain (LBP) is common after motor vehicle collisions (MVCs). A recent systematic literature review which identified 1,567 participants in three relevant studies reported that over half of adults involved in MVC develop new or worse LBP within 4 weeks. Rear-end collisions are the most common crash mechanism resulting in LBP.

Most LBP following a MVC is localized and not radicular in nature. In the absence of neurologic findings, it can be difficult to identify a specific cause of LBP. Common sources of pain include spinal and surrounding connective tissues that may have been injured by the sudden transfer of kinetic energy in the crash. Bones, joints (including the sacroiliac and facet joints), and lumbar intervertebral discs can also be sources of pain, but in the absence of an acute fracture, it may be difficult to know if they account for the new symptoms. LBP may predate the collision, and the reliability of patient-reported preexisting LBP is considered poor.

Serious pathology, although rare, can occur in MVCs, and the severity of the collision, loss of consciousness, sudden pain, and multiple traumas can alert responders at the scene to individuals who require emergency evaluation. Spinal fractures occur in less than 5% of all new LBP cases which present in primary care, the majority of which are caused by MVCs. About one-fifth of spinal fractures or dislocations are accompanied by spinal cord injuries. Lumbar radiculopathy in the MVC population is rare; its prevalence mirrors that in the non-MVC population.

A focused examination of the patient with LBP due to MVC includes inspection (with attention to obvious structural deformity or bruising on the painful area of the back), palpation of soft and bony tissues, assessment of active global trunk range of motion, and evaluation for neurologic loss and spinal and pelvic pathology. The patient should be asked if they experienced loss of consciousness and screened for other signs of concussion/traumatic brain injury and other musculoskeletal conditions (e.g. neck pain). For a patient such as this one who presents to the office several days later with LBP, the clinician should briefly screen for red flags which include: severe trauma, fever, unexplained weight loss, prior cancer, night pain, intravenous drug use, prolonged corticosteroid use, bowel or bladder dysfunction, saddle anesthesia, and severe neurologic deficits.

Imaging is unlikely to change initial management of patients with LBP after MVC in the absence of radicular symptoms and other red flags for serious or specific causes of LBP. Imaging not consistent with guideline recommendations may identify structural changes to the spine that were present prior to the MVC and therefore unlikely to be the cause of MVC-related pain. Such findings on imaging may unnecessarily worry the patient or clinician and may lead to clinical interventions to address specific findings that are most likely unrelated to MVC (e.g. pursuing an epidural steroid injection for disc bulge without progressive radiculopathy). Standard radiography or computerized tomography scans are appropriate when there is a suspicion of fracture, or symptoms are not improving with treatment. Concern of fracture is elevated for older patients, those with osteopenia or osteoporosis, and patients taking corticosteroids. Magnetic resonance imaging is appropriate for MVC patients with overt neurologic loss and for those with persistent radicular symptoms.

The majority of patients with MVC-related LBP are expected to recover within 4–10 weeks of the collision. Although the natural history of LBP after MVC is most often favorable, a third or more of patients report some level of persistent LBP at 12 months post-MVC, and a fifth report persistent pain at 7 years.

A full recovery of LBP after MVC may be affected by various biological, psychological, and social factors. The extent and severity of structural damage to the patient (e.g. spine or other fracture) may affect their recovery. The presence of additional musculoskeletal (e.g. neck pain) or other conditions (e.g. concussion) from MVC may also slow recovery. Additionally, psychological factors commonly influence the MVC patient's experience of pain, and comorbidities (both predating the MVC and concomitant with it) such as anxiety, depression, post-traumatic stress, and fear avoidance beliefs can complicate pain coping and delay recovery. Studies indicate that 10–20% of patients still suffer from post-traumatic neuropsychiatric sequelae at 1 year post-MVC, with as many as 30% suffering at 6 months. Social factors may also contribute to the patient's pain experience and influence recovery. For example, race/ethnicity differences have been observed in long-term MVC outcomes, with more Black than White patients developing chronic pain. This association may be influenced by race/ethnicity-related disparities in socioeconomic status and racial discrimination, including implicit bias of care providers.

Another social factor influencing the prognosis of LBP due to MVC is the potential impact of litigation. Though litigation is not thought to be a cause of pain, as with other psychosocial factors, it may influence recovery. Data suggest that reported pain is greater and recovery is poorer for patients who attribute fault to another or involve an attorney. Conversely, data also suggest a possible reduction in patients seeking care for pain following a MVC when there are fewer options for litigation, such as no-fault public insurance systems. The estimated risk of poor prognosis of LBP, related to psychological and social confounders, can be assessed on intake using a patient screening tool designed to stratify patients by risk of poor recovery, such as the short-form Örebro Musculoskeletal Pain or Keele STarT Back questionnaires.

Clinicians caring for patients with LBP due to MVC are encouraged to follow guideline recommendations for managing LBP in the absence of red flags. During the initial encounter, the clinician should provide education regarding the patient's condition and reassurance of a favorable prognosis. Self-care strategies, such as remaining active and not limiting physical activity due to pain, should be recommended as well during the first visit. Clinical practice guidelines recommend nonpharmacologic treatments (superficial heat, acupuncture, massage, and spinal manipulation) as first-line clinical treatments for acute LBP. Second-line treatments include pharmacologic agents, such as nonsteroidal anti-inflammatory drugs (NSAIDs) and muscle relaxants, which should be recommended after or concurrent with nonpharmacologic treatment. For persistent LBP, additional nonpharmacologic treatments are recommended, including exercise therapy, mindfulness-based stress reduction, and yoga.

Importantly, if the patient screening questionnaire indicates a high risk for developing chronic LBP, additional psychological support may be warranted (e.g. care from a behavioral health specialist or psychologically informed physical therapist). Furthermore, social determinants identified in screening such as low income, uninsured or underinsured status, food insecurity, and substance use may prompt linking the patient with a social worker or community health worker to support recovery.

In the scenario presented above, the patient is a 31-year-old with acute LBP of 1 week's duration following a MVC. He reports that there was no pain preceding, at the time of, or immediately following the collision. Pain began 1–2 days post-MVC and has become progressively worse. A focused exam should be performed as described above. The patient's report that his car was totaled raises concern for physical trauma and could warrant imaging. However, the patient did not experience immediate pain following the collision, he is young, and is presumably not taking corticosteroids, and he does not report any symptoms of neurologic deficit. Additionally, a correlation between the structural damage to a motor vehicle and the severity of injury to the driver is not supported in the literature, although patients can often incorrectly view the damage to their car as an indicator of the severity of injury to their bodies. If there are no concerning examination findings, the index of suspicion for fracture in this case is low, and imaging should therefore be deferred for at least 4 weeks pending a trial of therapy.

This patient is seeking help for his pain and has started to self-manage symptoms with an over the counter NSAID medication. While it is likely that he would benefit from a short course of this standard pharmacologic treatment, the patient may receive added benefit from a short course of first-line nonpharmacologic treatments such as acupuncture, moist heat, massage, or spinal manipulation. The patient should be informed of the correct dose of his particular NSAID and the potential harms of long-term NSAID use.

From a biological perspective, this patient's prognosis is favorable. Assuming red flags are excluded during history and examination, there is no apparent evidence of significant structural injury to patient from the MVC. Less is known of this patient's psychosocial profile, however, so administering a screening questionnaire for risk of poor recovery and asking follow-up questions regarding his emotional health and social determinants of health are recommended. His report that a friend drove him home from the crash is indicative of access to social support. However, sharing a photograph of his damaged vehicle with the examining clinician may indicate fear that, like his car, his back has sustained a significant structural injury, or a desire for validation of the seriousness of the situation. The photograph may also reflect the patient's sense of injustice after a crash that was out of his control, or a desire for the case to be documented for medicolegal reasons.

Most concerning is evidence that fear avoidance beliefs may be guiding how the patient is self-managing his LBP. This patient chose to rest at home in bed and on his couch rather than return to work or pursue active treatment. However, bed rest is not an effective treatment for acute LBP and can increase the likelihood the patient will develop persistent back-related pain or disability. These behaviors may indicate burgeoning kinesiophobia (fear of movement) and catastrophizing (considering a situation to be much worse than it actually is). Suspicion of fear avoidance beliefs is raised by his guarded gait and movements in the exam room.

Thus, even though he is expected to improve with time, there is concern that psychosocial factors, such as fear avoidance beliefs may limit or slow his recovery. Accordingly, excluding red flags, immediate validation of the patient's concerns, reassurance of a favorable prognosis, and education and compassionate encouragement that remaining active is not dangerous—and indeed is helpful—are important factors in optimizing this patient's prognosis. Reassuring phrases, such as "motion is lotion" and "hurt does not equal harm" may help the patient to incorporate this ideology. The patient should be encouraged specifically to return to his normal daily activities and exercise routine as tolerated, though he may wish to avoid intense exercise or stretching initially while the pain is severe. Physical therapy can provide graded exercise and address fear avoidance. The clinician should also recommend a return to work with time-limited activity modifications based upon his job requirements as needed.

Evidence of poor recovery on follow-up, despite active participation in physical treatments, should prompt consideration of referral for psychological and social health care. There is broad consensus among MVC experts that factors influencing recovery include preexisting psychosocial problems, level of social/workplace support, positive or negative expectations of recovery, catastrophic beliefs, resilience, coping skills, self-efficacy, and collaboration between the patient and members of the health care team. When recovery is poor, these factors should be assessed and addressed by behavioral health professionals to facilitate retraining patients' focus on recapturing their lives.

1. Over half of adults involved in MVCs develop new or worse LBP within 4 weeks, and a third report persistent pain at 12 months.

2. History and exam of those with LBP after a MVC should include assessing psychosocial comorbidities and social determinants of health. Imaging should only be ordered when there is suspicion of fracture or pain is not improving after 4 weeks of conservative treatment.

3. Up to a third of patients involved in a collision suffer from post-traumatic neuropsychiatric sequelae at 6 months. Patient screening tools designed to identify psychosocial risk factors for persistent disability should be utilized on intake.

4. After ruling out serious pathology, the clinician should provide education and reassurance of a favorable prognosis and encourage appropriate physical activity. Established first- and second-line clinical care protocols should be followed if pain persists.

Further reading

1. Nolet PS, Emary PC, Kristman VL, Murnaghan K, Zeegers MP, Freeman MD. Exposure to a motor vehicle collision and the risk of future back pain: a systematic review and meta-analysis. Accid Anal Prev. 2020;142:105546.

2. Smits EJ, Gane EM, Brakenridge CL, Andrews NE, Johnston V. Expert consensus and perspectives on recovery following road traffic crashes: a Delphi study. Disabil Rehabil. 2022;44(13):3122–3131.

3. Williams CM, Henschke N, Maher CG, et al. Red flags to screen for vertebral fracture in patients presenting with low-back pain. Cochrane Database Syst Rev. 2023;(1).

4. Chou R, Qaseem A, Snow V, et al. Diagnosis and treatment of low back pain: a joint clinical practice guideline from the American College of Physicians and the American Pain Society. Ann Intern Med. 2007;147(7):478–491.

5. Qaseem A, Wilt TJ, McLean RM, Forciea MA; Clinical Guidelines Committee of the American College of P. Noninvasive treatments for acute, subacute, and chronic low back pain: a clinical practice guideline from the American College of Physicians. Ann Intern Med. 2017;166(7):514–530.

20 "I Was Hurt at Work, and I'll Get Hurt Again if I Go Back.": Back Pain and Workplace Injury

Kristina Barber, Christopher J. Standaert, Rachel Brakke Holman

A 36-year-old presents with back pain following an injury at work. The patient works in construction and had been with a new employer for 2 months before the injury. They note that 4 months ago they were carrying one end of a large beam, when the worker holding the other end let go suddenly. Low back pain occurred immediately. The patient went to an urgent care center that day and was given medications. Although initially improving with chiropractic care and physical therapy, an MRI was performed showing "disc desiccation and a broad-based bulge" at L4/L5. The pain has lessened steadily, and the patient is able to walk and function at home without pain. However, they have not gone back to work. When asked about this, the patient responds, "If I go back, I'm

just going to get hurt again." The patient is also
not going to the gym for routine exercise due
to the same concern. There is paperwork from
the worker's compensation carrier sitting on the
exam table next to the patient.

What do you do now?

Low back pain (LBP) affects the majority of Americans sometime during their working years. Although it is commonly taught that up to 90% of patients with acute LBP show prompt recovery and return to work within 1–3 months of injury, the reality is most people with LBP have recurrent pain within 1 year and only about one-third fully recover at 12 months. In the workers' compensation setting, LBP claims remain open for about one-third of patients at 3 months. This partly explains why LBP, despite having a positive natural history for many, is the second most common reason for short-term disability claims and the most common reason for long-term disability claims in the United States. Although this population can be challenging to treat, active intervention to narrow this discordance falls in large part on treating providers, particularly with early efforts to help patients remain active and working. A conservative yet holistic approach identifying and addressing associated biopsychosocial factors has been proven effective for enhancing return to work.

Work-related LBP is often nonspecific with no red flag symptoms. Absent concerns for significant pathology, such as a fracture, or neurologic concerns, imaging of the lumbar spine tends to show expected age-related changes and is unlikely to change an initial recommendation of conservative care. Although the injury may be pathologically minor, the psychosocial overlay can magnify the level of disability. Coping with LBP has more to do with these psychosocial confounders of daily life inside and/or outside the workplace rather than the magnitude of pain itself. Most injured workers will improve and return to work, so identifying risk factors for deviation from this expected pattern is important.

Predictive factors can be broken down into health-related, work-related, and systems-related. Health-related factors predicting failure to return to work include severity of pain, premorbid depression, low self-confidence, catastrophizing, fear avoidance, and not returning to work within 6 months. Fear avoidance beliefs are cognitions and fears about potential for physical activity to produce pain and harm. Catastrophizing is the summation of cognitive and emotional responses to pain leading to magnification, rumination, and helplessness. Patients who display catastrophizing have higher pain levels, worse function, and more psychological distress than those who do not. Work-related factors that negatively predict return to work include the lack of availability of light or modified duty, job tenure of less than 1 year, and physical work demands. Additionally, poor coworker relationships and poor job satisfaction are related to a lower probability of returning to work. Systems-related factors include compensation and litigation. Return to work is less likely if there is attorney involvement or interaction with disability compensation programs.

Patients can present with varied emotions including anger, depression, anxiety, fear, catastrophizing, and loss of identity. Presence of depression or anxiety predicts higher pain, decreased function, and the transition from an acute to chronic phase of disease. Those with pre-injury depression are 33% less likely to return to work and may take up to twice as long to return. When out of work, patients can also develop an altered sense of self which can lead to loss of self-confidence, isolation, substance abuse, and even suicide. While not a formal psychiatric diagnosis, anger is a neglected but important emotion in the pain experience. Patients experiencing anger are prone to denying this emotion due to societal norms which discourage harboring or expressing angry feelings. As they never appropriately acknowledge or express their anger, they are unlikely to resolve this emotion. Rather, they internalize the feeling and indirectly express it through pain, depression, or more socially legitimate complaints.

Delving into the patient's coping strategies can be illuminating. This can be done with simple questioning or with a tool like the Coping Strategies Questionnaire. Active coping aimed at controlling pain and function is linked to positive affect, improved adjustment, and decreased depression. Typically, patients who adopt this strategy return to work quickly. On the other hand, passive coping (excessive rest, activity avoidance, hoping, and praying) relinquishes control of pain to others and is linked to increased depression and pain. Patients who utilize passive coping may also develop fear avoidance or catastrophizing mentalities. This behavior has been described as the single most important risk factor for poor response to pain-relieving interventions, lack of return to work, and progression to chronic pain.

Providers must shift from identifying and treating any presumed structural source of LBP to focusing on factors limiting the patient's return to work. Those who do not return to work face the reality that unemployment is strongly correlated with all-cause mortality including cardiovascular disease and suicide. Clarifying a patient's expectations of care can help providers understand belief structures, barriers, and social constructs that may be obstacles to improvement. Providers can use this to create opportunity for education when expectations deviate from what is medically indicated.

Providers should de-medicalize the patient's beliefs by reframing LBP as a normal part of life and a condition that can be remedied with conservative treatment rather than with advanced imaging, invasive procedures, surgery, or narcotics. This reframing requires balance with the fact that patients need validation of their suffering. Providers should delve into the emotions associated with the pain experience, specifically asking about those mentioned previously, as a mental health referral may be indicated. Cognitive behavioral therapy (CBT) and acceptance and commitment therapy (ACT) can reframe negative automatic cognitions like fear and catastrophizing and lead to improved pain and function. Social isolation can be addressed by encouraging reengagement with friends, family, and coworkers. Social workers and vocational rehabilitation counselors can assist with resources for community and work reengagement. For workers with LBP, provider attitude makes a difference. Emphasis on using optimism, positivity, and reassurance can improve pain intensity, reduce situational pain catastrophizing, and buffer fear of movement. Motivational interviewing can also be utilized.

Providers need to clearly communicate their recommendation that the patient should return to work. Even when chronic disability has begun, a clear decree can be influential. Simply put, workers specifically instructed to return to work are more likely to return to work. Counseling on cardiovascular and muscular deconditioning leading to decline in aerobic fitness and endurance should be provided to set expectations of the process of reconditioning. Recommendations should include a graded reintroduction of physical activity, whether this be patient-directed (i.e. increasing daily walking time or distance), with physical therapy, or ideally both. Therapy can include engaging in specific movement patterns or feared activities to improve fear avoidance and functional disability as well.

When speaking about return to work, providers should ask about the specific duties involved in their patient's job. This adds to the therapeutic relationship and allows providers to give specific work restrictions and address how to avoid reinjury at work. For most patients with mild, nonspecific LBP interfering with work, physicians should avoid removing patients from work. It is clearly more beneficial to recommend temporary "light duty" or modified duty which restricts the number of hours of work allowed and/or specific work activities. While the patient engages in conservative treatment, including physical therapy, light duty is a way to limit developing the psychosocial comorbidities associated with being out of work. If modified duties are not available or a patient has plateaued with their conservative therapy, work hardening or work conditioning programs are viable alternatives to short-term disability or forced inactivity. Work hardening is an individualized, interdisciplinary, job-specific program to assist with return to work that uses simulated work activities and graded increases in activity to restore function and vocation ability physically and psychosocially.

Lastly, with regards to follow up, if patients identify risk factors described previously, an emphasis on closer follow up can be utilized to monitor for progression to subacute and chronic pain, functional disability, and delayed return to work. Follow-up should include eventual discussion and explicit recommendation of returning to work. Alternatively, for patients without such factors, leaving follow-up to patient discretion can help reduce health care use and de-medicalize their condition.

In this case, the patient is a young heavy-duty construction worker who has been hurt on the job. After 4 months, their pain has improved with conservative care so that they can perform daily tasks with ease, but they have not returned to work. This patient is nearing the 6-month time point at which their chance of return to work declines significantly. They are physically deconditioned and have associated psychological comorbidities including fear avoidance and catastrophizing that have not been addressed. Avoiding activity, including returning to the gym and work, due to fear specifically of the uncontextualized "disc desiccation and bulge" on MRI is related to their catastrophizing that activity will cause another injury. This patient has had limited follow-up with no clear instruction to return to work and is beginning a disability application.

While this patient would have benefited from earlier identification of risk factors, better understanding of job duties, recommendation of light duty, and closer follow-up, progression to chronic pain and disability can be modified. This appointment would be a good time to zoom out, reframe pain in relation to function, and delve into coping strategies. Next steps would include recommendation of graded increase in activity and discussion of exploring light or modified duty opportunities at their work. The fear avoidant behavior needs to be addressed. The MRI findings should be placed in context, as they are quite normal for age and not indicative of or predictive of a significant injury. It is important to provide reassurance that it is both safe and essential that they get back to the gym, initially with low impact cardiovascular activity and exercise as guided by their physical therapist. Exercise ultimately has to progress to work- and life-specific tasks. There is no indication for interventional care or surgical consultation here, and the patient needs an understanding that they can continue to improve from this point and get back to work. If they are relying on passive forms of short-term relief like manipulation or rest, these need to be discouraged. Referral to a psychologist to address fear, anger, or similar emotions and to discuss pacing can be helpful. Referral to a work-hardening program to improve physical capacity specifically for work is an option for those with particularly strenuous or technically demanding jobs.

Although the patient in this case is not defined as being of a specific gender or ethnicity, these factors do need to be considered when caring for injured workers. In general, women or those of an ethnocultural minority face greater challenges in returning to work after an injury. African Americans and those of lower socioeconomic status show higher rates of pain, psychological distress, and disability after closure of workers compensation claims. If the patient in this case was a woman, they would likely be faced with bias toward their role and capacity in a male-dominated industry. All of those otherwise marginalized may face lower levels of trust, greater vulnerability, and more difficulty obtaining appropriate accommodations. Individuals with less financial resources or social support often have difficulty with economic sustainability while off of work following injury, lessening their options for achieving a successful return. A patient who has experienced prior trauma or discrimination may have distinct adverse reactions to injury or perceptions of a hostile work environment. Those in any of these situations may experience more fear and distress. The cultural context of a given patient is also associated with distinctive belief structures and social and family roles. All patients need to be heard and to have their unique experience factored into any treatment plan. They also may need assistance with managing the additional barriers that they face to achieve optimal outcomes.

1. For most patients, LBP is a chronic, recurrent disorder, which requires providers to think proactively about managing patients over time.
2. Coping with disability due to LBP has more to do with psychosocial factors rather than the magnitude of pain itself.
3. Early identification and management of risk factors including depression, fear avoidance, catastrophizing, and social isolation can improve rates of returning to work.
4. Providers should de-medicalize by reframing LBP as a normal part of life and a condition that can be remedied with conservative treatment.
5. While patients engage in conservative treatment including physical therapy, light duty should be recommended to promote return to work and mitigate associated psychosocial comorbidities.

Further reading

1. Aanesen F, Berg R, Løchting I, et al. Motivational interviewing and return to work for people with musculoskeletal disorders: a systematic mapping review. J Occup Rehabil. 2021;31(1):63–71. doi:10.1007/s10926-020-09892-0.
2. Dasinger LK, Krause N, Thompson PJ, Brand RJ, Rudolph L. Doctor proactive communication, return-to-work recommendation, and duration of disability after a workers' compensation low back injury. J Occup Environ Med. 2001;43(6):515–525. doi:10.1097/00043764-200106000-00001.
3. Meints SM, Edwards RR. Evaluating psychosocial contributions to chronic pain outcomes. Prog Neuropsychopharmacol Biol Psychiatry. 2018;87(Pt B):168–182. doi:10.1016/j.pnpbp.2018.01.017.
4. Shaw WS, Nelson CC, Woiszwillo MJ, Gaines B, Peters SE. Early return to work has benefits for relief of back pain and functional recovery after controlling for multiple confounds. J Occup Environ Med. 2018;60(10):901–910. doi:10.1097/JOM.0000000000001380.
5. Steele J, Bruce-Low S, Smith D. A reappraisal of the deconditioning hypothesis in low back pain: review of evidence from a triumvirate of research methods on specific lumbar extensor deconditioning. Curr Med Res Opin. 2014;30(5):865–911. doi:10.1185/03007995.2013.875465.

21 "I Just Had Surgery, but I Hurt Again.": Back and Leg Pain 4 Months after Back Surgery

Alex Watson, Christopher J. Standaert

Your patient comes in with recurrent back and leg pain. You saw them last year for a similar problem. Workup at that time revealed a disc protrusion at L5/S1 with compromise of the right S1 nerve root in the spinal canal. Due to persistent pain after physical therapy, medications, and an epidural steroid injection, the patient underwent a microdiscectomy by a local spine surgeon 4 months ago. Initially things went well, and the leg pain resolved. A few visits with physical therapy seemed helpful. However, starting about 2 months ago, your patient noted some recurrence of low back pain. This came on over several days and was followed by progressive right leg pain. At this point, the pain is similar to what the patient experienced before surgery. They complain of pain in the back and buttock and paresthesia into the right posterior thigh and calf. It is hard for them to walk briskly for more than 30 minutes, and the stretching from physical therapy now results in leg pain.

What do you do now?

Treating patients with a history of spine surgery requires consideration of issues that are distinct from those in patients with no prior surgery. Surgery often involves damage to or removal of structures that play a role in stabilizing the spine or the implantation of material that alters normal mobility of the spine. Consequences can arise from either of these factors or from the direct trauma and invasive nature of surgery in general. When thinking through the potential consequences of surgery, issues of instability, infection, scarring, re-herniation of a disc, progressive degeneration or collapse of a disc, and problems at levels adjacent to the surgery all have to be considered. Bleeding (e.g. an epidural hematoma) and dural fluid leak are additional concerns in the acute postoperative setting. For the most part, patients with a history of spine surgery are excluded from the majority of studies of low back pain (LBP), which complicates our understanding of treating these patients when subsequent problems arise.

Discectomy is the standard surgical approach to treat a lumbar disc herniation with a radiculopathy. There are variations in how the spine is accessed, but the surgery involves an incision in the low back and often removal of bone from the back of the vertebra (a laminotomy or laminectomy) in order to access the spinal canal. Disc material is then removed from the epidural space, freeing up the affected nerve root. Patients often have a rapid improvement in symptoms, and the majority of patients have successful outcomes, although persistent symptoms, to some degree, are common. Approximately 10% of individuals will suffer perioperative complications, and 7% will require reoperation within 1 year. Within 10 years following surgery, approximately 25% of individuals will require another spine surgery. Smoking, comorbid diabetes, depression, and disability are risk factors for recurrent back and/or leg pain.

When a patient presents with recurrent radicular pain following a discectomy, a clinician will need to work through a differential diagnosis that includes recurrent herniation of the same disc, a novel disc herniation, infection (discitis/osteomyelitis), spinal instability, epidural fibrosis, and arachnoiditis (see Table 21.1). These conditions are often lumped under the term "failed back syndrome," but this is an unhelpful, nonspecific term with an implication that somehow it is the patient, or their back, that has failed. This is both untrue and inaccurate. Diagnostic specificity is highly preferred.

TABLE 21.1 Differential Diagnosis of Recurrent Low Back and Leg Pain After Discectomy

Recurrent or New Disc Herniation

Spinal Instability or Spondylolisthesis

Infection (Discitis, Vertebral Osteomyelitis)

Epidural Fibrosis

Arachnoiditis

Bleeding/Epidural Hematoma (acute)

Spinal fluid leak (acute)

Research suggests that nearly 25% of patients with recurring LBP following discectomy will have a recurrent disc herniation. A large (6+ mm in width) initial defect in the annulus fibrosis that is not repaired in the initial discectomy increases the risk of recurrent herniation. Alternatively, those with diffuse degenerative change of the spine or those with prior fusion are vulnerable to new disc herniation and other complications postoperatively. In the postoperative setting, these are treated much as any acute disc herniation with predominantly nonsurgical care (see chapter 5). On the whole, repeat surgery for discs that have re-herniated have lower success rates than primary surgeries.

Spinal instability can result from a combination of post-surgical changes and degenerative changes. A discectomy can involve significant resection of bone or ligamentous structures, which can increase the risk of postoperative instability. In some cases, this leads to a vertebra translating inappropriately on top of the one below it (a spondylolisthesis—see chapter 9). Symptoms can include LBP, radicular pain, and a feeling of the back "giving way" or shifting with movement.

Postoperative infection of the vertebrae (osteomyelitis) and/or the disc (discitis) is a serious complication of discectomy. Often, pain begins insidiously and may progress over weeks to months. Symptoms typically include local pain, tenderness to palpation, spasms in adjacent muscles, and potentially fever or malaise. Inflammatory markers, such as erythrocyte sedimentation rate (ESR) and C-reactive protein (CRP) are almost always elevated.

Patients inconsistently have fever, and, therefore, the absence of fever does not rule out infection. If the infection extends into the epidural space, additional symptoms can arise due to spinal cord or cauda equina compression, including new onset weakness or sensory deficits in the legs, saddle anesthesia, and bowel/bladder dysfunction. Discitis occurs with a frequency of about 0.1–4% following all spinal procedures and after about one in 400 microdiscectomies. Postoperative discitis accounts for about 25% of all cases of discitis. Discitis/osteomyelitis is frequently associated with destruction of the vertebral endplates, disc inflammation, associated abscesses, and other related findings on imaging (see chapter 15 for further discussion of discitis).

Epidural fibrosis or epidural scarring is a risk after any spinal surgical intervention, as the body responds to the invasive procedure. Scar formation is a normal part of healing, so some scarring is expected. In fact, the invasiveness correlates with the occurrence of the fibrosis (i.e., the extent of scarring is less in a single-level surgery than a multilevel procedure). Most patients with recurrent LBP will have some degree of epidural fibrosis, although the severity of fibrosis is poorly correlated to the level of pain. Diagnostically, magnetic resonance imaging (MRI) of the lumbar spine with and without intravenous contrast will demonstrate enhancing fibrotic material in the epidural space. This enhancement helps distinguish fibrosis/scar, which is highly vascular, from disc material, which is not vascular. If the enhancing fibrotic tissue surrounds or otherwise affects the nerve roots, it may potentially be associated with radicular pain (see Figure 21.1).

Arachnoiditis is inflammation of the arachnoid mater layer of the meninges overlying the spinal cord and nerve roots in the cerebrospinal fluid (CSF). In the context of discectomy, arachnoiditis occurs with intraoperative dural tears. This trauma leads to inflammatory cell infiltration and fibrosis in the subarachnoid space, which causes subsequent entrapment and adherence of lumbosacral nerve roots and/or the cauda equina. On MRI, the nerve roots can appear clumped or may adhere to the dura, leaving the nerve roots seemingly absent from the intra-dural space (see Figure 21.2). Given the number of nerves potentially involved, arachnoiditis may clinically mimic lumbar spinal stenosis or a disc process resulting in root compression or cause cauda equina syndrome in severe cases. Not all patients who develop radiographic arachnoiditis have clinical problems, but those

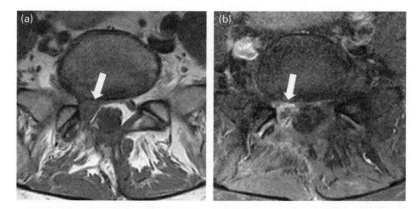

FIGURE 21.1. T1 weighted axial MRI images at L5/S1, pre- (a) and post-intravenous (b) contrast administration, of a patient with right leg pain following a microdiscectomy. Note the dark material on the patient's right (a) in the region of the S1 nerve root (arrow). In (b), following intravenous contrast administration, that same area is white or "enhanced," indicating significant vascularity. The S1 nerve (dark oval within the white) can now be seen surrounded by the enhancing epidural fibrosis (scar tissue, arrow).

Figure 21.1a. Pre-contrast.

Figure 21.1b. Post-contrast.

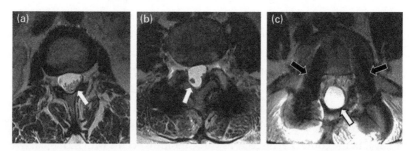

FIGURE 21.2. T2 weighted axial MRI images from a patient with symptomatic arachnoiditis following a lumbar spinal fusion complicated by intra-operative dural tear.

Figure 21.2a. Image through L1/L2 showing normal nerve root anatomy within the dura (arrow).

Figure 21.2b. Image through L3/L4 showing clumping of the nerve roots within the dura (arrow).

Figure 21.2c. Image through L4/L5 showing peripheralization of the nerve roots with none readily visible within the cerebrospinal fluid (white arrow). Signal change from pedicle screws is seen on either side of the dura (black arrows).

who are affected can have mono- or poly-radicular pain, weakness, numbness, or bowel or bladder dysfunction. The pain can be severe and highly disabling. There are no pathognomonic symptoms associated with the onset of arachnoiditis, which typically occurs in the acute to immediately postoperative time period. In addition to a surgical violation of the dura, arachnoiditis can occur from an intradural infection or chemical irritation from substances that are instilled or otherwise enter the dura.

Returning to the patient presented above, the initial evaluation begins as any typical assessment of pain, carefully determining factors such as the onset, palliative/precipitating interventions, and the quality, severity, and timing of the pain. In this case, the LBP recurred 2 months after surgery, developed over several days, and was followed by progressive right leg pain. The symptoms are persistent and similar to those which the patient experienced before surgery, with pain in the back and buttock and paresthesia into the right posterior thigh and calf. These make it hard for the patient to walk briskly or stretch. These suggest recurrent involvement of the right S1 root.

Questions about red flag symptoms are critical here, including inquiring about new saddle anesthesia, bowel/bladder dysfunction, constitutional symptoms (such as fever, malaise, and weight loss), and pain that worsens substantially when supine. Finally, the history should include screening for depression and new psychological stressors, as pain perception can be augmented by mood disorders or significant acute stress.

The physical exam begins with inspection of the prior incision site for signs of infection, sequelae of poor healing, drainage from the prior surgical site, or subcutaneous fluid. Palpate around the incision site for focal pain, mass, or fluctuance. Perform a general neuromuscular exam of the lower extremities to evaluate for new sensorimotor deficits that would be suggestive of acute nerve compression/injury, which includes gait, strength, reflexes, and sensation assessment. It is helpful to have documentation of the neurologic exam preoperatively so new neurologic loss can be distinguished from deficits that were previously present.

Serum labs are integral to screening, as discitis is a "cannot-miss" diagnosis. Obtain a complete blood count (CBC), ESR, and CRP to identify signs of inflammation that would be suggestive of infection. Elevations in the ESR and CRP are seen in about 90% of patients with discitis, while leukocytosis is less common. Initial imaging should include standing lumbar-spine X-rays with flexion and extension views. This basic workup is expedient and inexpensive, and these results help to screen for infection and spinal instability as the etiology of pain. If inflammatory markers are elevated, or there is evidence of infection on X-ray such as destruction of the vertebrae, an MRI of the lumbar spine with and without contrast should be obtained. Patients with confirmed or high suspicion of an infection, instability, or new neurological loss should be referred to their surgeon or otherwise evaluated emergently.

This patient does not have clear emergent symptoms or findings (although the laboratory studies and X-rays described above are necessary). Due to the significant leg pain and functional limitations, however, an MRI with and without intravenous contrast is indicated to look for evidence of a recurrent disc herniation or epidural fibrosis, among other potential causes of the leg pain. In this case, the MRI appears as in Figure 21.1, showing epidural fibrosis around the S1 root without a recurrent disc herniation. This fits with the history of initial recovery from surgery followed by the gradual return of pain over a few months. There is no role for repeat surgery in this setting, and this patient's management should focus on nonsurgical, noninterventional options. Although the visualized scar may not resolve over time (it may reduce), the patient's symptoms can improve and generally be managed effectively.

There are no high-level data to guide management of this condition (epidural fibrosis). Counsel the patient on the need for time to allow for gradual improvement of their symptoms, as this may take 6–12 months and will likely be incomplete. Medications for neuropathic pain, such as serotonin-norepinephrine reuptake inhibitors (SNRIs), tricyclic antidepressants (TCAs), or gabapentin/pregabalin, should be considered and may potentially improve symptoms and permit greater participation in physical therapy (PT). SNRIs or TCAs may have added benefit in treating comorbid mood disorders, and TCAs administered in the evening can improve sleep. Nonsteroidal, anti-inflammatory medications or oral steroids can also be considered. None of these medications are well-studied in this setting.

PT can be helpful to guide patients in their recovery. Often there is significant "dural tension" on the affected nerve, meaning that it is tethered at the area of scar and can be very sensitive to stretch or traction. Hence, excessive stretching of the hamstrings or attempts to mobilize the nerve through physical maneuvers should be avoided when the nerve is highly symptomatic. These can be done more effectively if the pain and sensitivity of the nerve are less acute. Patients may need to reduce tension through the nerve by walking with a shorter stride length and avoiding walking uphill, bending forward at the waist, or stretching their hamstrings. If activity restriction, medication, and gentle mobilization are effective in managing the pain (which often takes 3–12 months), patients can then gradually progress their activity. Although occasionally used, there is no evidence that epidural steroid injections are effective in this patient population. Surgery to remove the scar tissue is largely ineffective and best avoided. There is no identified "curative" treatment for this condition.

Pain recurrence after microdiscectomy is an unfortunate but not infrequent occurrence. Physicians must rule out infection or acute nerve compression early in the workup. Screening for depression is crucial, as it may worsen pain perception, or the return of pain may have precipitated worsening mental health. In the absence of emergent findings, physicians should provide reassurance and multimodal pain control to facilitate participation in physical therapy for long-term benefit.

KEY POINTS

1. Postoperative pain after lumbar microdiscectomy is relatively common—approximately 10% of patients suffer complications, and 7% require reoperation within 2 months.
2. Given the frequency and potential severity of postoperative complications, all of those with persistent, progressive, or severe symptoms following a microdiscectomy (or other spine surgery) warrant prompt diagnostic evaluation.
3. Screen patients with postoperative pain with basic labs of CBC, ESR, and CRP for infection and standing lumbar spine AP, lateral, and flexion/extension X-rays. MRI of the lumbar spine with and without intravenous contrast may be indicated.
4. Infection, new neurologic deficit, and instability warrant referral to the surgeon or emergent evaluation.

5. For nonemergent cases, reassurance is critical, as recurrent pain and disability present a significant psychologic burden. Screen for new stressors, depression, and sleep disorders that may worsen pain.

Further reading
1. Huang W, Han Z, Liu J, Yu L, Yu X. Risk factors for recurrent lumbar disc herniation: a systematic review and meta-analysis. Medicine. 2016;95(2):e2378. https://doi.org/10.1097/MD.0000000000002378.
2. Sebaaly A, Lahoud MJ, Rizkallah M, Kreichati G, Kharrat K. Etiology, evaluation, and treatment of failed back surgery syndrome. Asian Spine J. 2018;12(3):574–585. https://doi.org/10.4184/asj.2018.12.3.574.
3. Bosscher HA, Heavner JE. Incidence and severity of epidural fibrosis after back surgery: an endoscopic study. Pain Pract. 2010;10:18–24. https://doi.org/10.1111/j.1533-2500.2009.00311.x.
4. Tsuchida R, Sumitani M, Azuma K, et al. A novel technique using magnetic resonance imaging in the supine and prone positions for diagnosing lumbar adhesive arachnoiditis: a preliminary study. Pain Pract. 2020;20: 34–43. https://doi.org/10.1111/papr.12822.
5. Papadopoulos EC, Girardi FP, Sandhu HS, et al. Outcome of revision discectomies following recurrent lumbar disc herniation. Spine. 2006 June 1;31(13):1473–1476. doi: 10.1097/01.brs.0000219872.43318.7a.

22 "I Can't Run without Pain.": Low Back Pain While Training for the Boston Marathon

Katharine Smolinski, Mark A. Harrast

A 24-year-old female presents with a complaint of relatively acute left low back pain (LBP). She notes she has been training to run the Boston Marathon in a couple months, which will be her first marathon. She had been active and running intermittently prior to starting to train for the marathon but has had no formal training in track or distance running. Yoga was her predominant exercise otherwise. She has been trying to push her training mileage to prepare for the marathon but has been limited recently by pain in her lower left lumbar to sacral area. It hurts to run. There is no real radiation into her leg. She is better with less activity but has been trying to maintain her training despite the pain. She has no history of LBP but did injure her left ankle playing frisbee a few years ago. On exam, she has a BMI of 19.1, her gait is a bit antalgic, and she is neurologically intact.

What do you do now?

Running-related injuries tend to be insidious in onset, multifactorial in origin, and often involve a component of overuse. Risk factors for injury include personal characteristics of the runner (anatomical and biomechanical factors) and improper training (increasing training volume or intensity too quickly and inadequate rest). Total weekly mileage and prior history of running-related injury are two important predictors for risk of injury in the runner. Increased risk begins at 19 miles per week and in runners with less than 3 years of experience.

The differential diagnosis for LBP in the runner is broad. A running athlete can present with the common sources of LBP as well as more running related etiologies. Runners may have LBP that is relatively nonspecific from a structural perspective but is generally thought to be related to imbalances/deficits in musculoskeletal function that adversely impact or overly stress the lumbar region. An example would be weakness or instability related to prior ankle injury that leads to an abnormal running gait, eventually stressing the lumbar region (which may play a role in our patient in this case). Gluteal muscle or hip rotator tears occur in runners and can cause buttock pain. Proximal hamstring tendinopathy is a common source of distal buttock pain in the aging runner. Spondylolysis (a stress injury to the pars interarticularis) is a common cause of LBP in adolescent athletes, in general (see chapter 25). Runners of any age are also prone to bone stress injuries (BSI) in the femur, pelvis, or sacrum. Finally, the hip can refer to the posterior pelvis, and thus hip pathology (impingement in a younger patient and arthritis in an older patient are two of the more common etiologies) should be included on the differential diagnosis of buttock pain.

The purpose of the history in a runner with LBP is to identify individual risk factors for injury and to rule out any "red flags" that would warrant more aggressive evaluation and intervention. In addition to the history one might obtain for anyone with acute LBP, the clinician should inquire about historical factors related to bone health, cues to energy balance, and a specific running history. See Table 22.1 for a detailed intake history. For the female runner, it is important to ascertain age of menarche (primary amenorrhea: menarche > age 15) and regularity of menstrual cycles (oligomenorrhea: menses <6–8/year), as disorders in menstruation may alert the provider to related energy deficiency, which suggests risk for BSI.

TABLE 22.1 Medical and Training History for the Injured Runner

Factor	Additional Questions to Ask
Medical History	
Chronic medical conditions	Low bone mineral density, inflammatory bowel disease, celiac disease, endocrinologic disorders, chronic medications?
Menstrual history	Age of menarche, frequency of menses, last menstrual period?
Prior fractures	Traumatic or stress-induced?
Prior running injuries	What were they, when did they occur, what was the treatment? Any residual pain from prior injury?
Dietary habits	Approximate caloric intake, dietary restrictions, history of disordered eating?
Weight	Typical running weight? Does it fluctuate significantly when running more?
Training History	
Running experience	How long have you been running? Recreational, competitive, or elite level?
Running goals	Upcoming race, weight loss, overall health, social outlet?
Running load	Weekly distance, runs per week, speed intensity?
Changes in training	Running volume, frequency, intensity terrain, or shoes?
Current training program	Structured program? Do you have a coach? Running with a partner or a group?
Cross-training and other exercise	What activities and what frequency?
Typical running surfaces	Beveled roads, same route all the time?
Footwear And Equipment	
Shoes	Type of shoe and how did you choose it? How long have you been wearing that shoe?
Orthotics	What kind, how long have you used them, why did you start using them?
Other equipment	Armbands, water bottles, hydration belt, strollers?

In addition to the standard neuromusculoskeletal evaluation in any patient presenting with LBP, the assessment of the injured runner should include a basic functional evaluation of the kinetic chain, incorporating both static and dynamic testing. The "kinetic chain" is the sequence of movements across a series of joints leading to an intended action. Running is basically a series of single-leg squats. It can be enlightening to examine the runner as they perform both double- and single-leg squats in the office, while evaluating for dynamic hip stability and deficits in neuromuscular control (see Figure 22.1). This may translate to how the runner controls their gait while running a distance over time. Ideally, the runner can maintain good sagittal

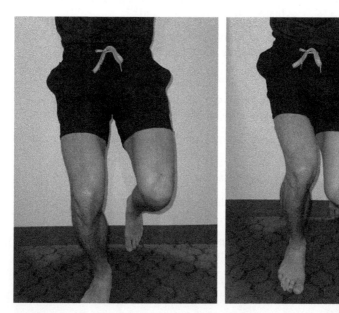

FIGURE 22.1. Functional examination of the runner. The runner is descending during the eccentric phase of the single-leg squat. The runner on the left (A) is demonstrating good neuromuscular control at the pelvis/hip. The runner on the right (B) is demonstrating medial knee movement of the standing leg with femoral adduction and internal rotation, as well as over pronation distally, and contralateral pelvic hip drop, all suggesting poor lumbo-pelvic-hip neuromuscular control. Lack of dynamic stability suggests biomechanical insufficiencies in the stance phase of the running gait. This pelvic instability can produce additional stress on the lumbar spine (i.e. the next proximal segment) which ultimately can contribute to pain. Deficits detected in this controlled, non-fatigued state, are likely to be amplified when fatigue develops during training.

alignment of the leg and a level position of the pelvis with a single-leg squat. Frequently, dynamic weakness presents as medial deviation of the ipsilateral knee and lowering of the contralateral hip. A full running gait evaluation can often be obtained through physical therapy to assess for common biomechanical faults (see Table 22.2). However, this should be delayed if there are concerns about BSI or worsening pain with continued running.

In the absence of red flag symptoms or bony point tenderness, it is often reasonable to proceed with conservative management of LBP and defer imaging pending progress with treatment. However, if the runner's training goal is upcoming, or if there is any concern for BSI, it may be helpful to image early in order to direct management most appropriately and efficiently. In addition to the standard imaging evaluation for any patient with

TABLE 22.2   **Common Biomechanical Factors in Running Gait Evaluations**

Initial Contact:

- Foot strike pattern—while there is no common optimal foot strike pattern, observation of patterns can indicate where the body may be experiencing more stress

Midstance:

- From posterior view—look at the knee "window" or amount of light visible between the knees
- From anterior view—look at the direction of the patella in order to determine excessive hip adduction, femoral internal rotation, or knee valgus
- Look for contralateral pelvic drop, which is a sign of insufficient hip abduction and external rotation strength of the stance leg
- Look for trunk lean toward stance leg, which is also a sign of lateral hip muscle weakness of stance leg

Toe-Off:

- Observe dynamic leg alignment (the line connecting ankle, knee, and hip)

Full Gait Cycle:

- Look for excessive hip and knee excursion from initial contact, which may indicate the runner has insufficient strength to stabilize against impact forces

LBP, magnetic resonance imaging (MRI) is indicated when evaluating a runner with a possible bone stress injury. As these injuries often occur in the sacrum, ilium, or femur, this requires a pelvis MRI, which may also show musculotendinous injuries if present. MRI is the most sensitive and specific imaging modality for BSI (see Table 22.3).

In this particular case, we encounter a young, female runner with relatively acute LBP without radicular symptoms, in the context of increased training load. She has a low normal BMI without any known chronic medical conditions, a prior history of ankle injury, limited previous running experience without structured training, and a time-specific goal. She is neurologically intact with no red flag symptoms. Although there are a number of potential causes of sacral pain, the history of increasing mileage in a novice distance runner with a time-specific goal and notable sacral tenderness suggests a sacral BSI. Proceeding with more history to elucidate this runner's bone health, as noted above, is important. One question that always needs to be answered when evaluating an injured runner is: "Is it safe for the runner to continue running?" If our concern for sacral BSI is validated, the answer is clearly "no." Thus, to confirm our suspicion, an MRI of the pelvis or sacrum is indicated, as it will help us counsel the patient more assuredly about how/when to return to running.

The sacrum is a cancellous, or trabecular, bone. BSI of cancellous bone is suggestive of an insufficiency fracture and thus low bone density (likely compounded by running training errors). Risk factors for low bone mineral density (BMD) include energy imbalance (energy out (exercise)> energy in (nutrition/calories)), chronic malabsorptive disorders (celiac disease, inflammatory bowel disease), medication exposures (corticosteroids), and endocrinologic abnormalities. It is important to consider the impact of

TABLE 22.3 **Imaging Modalities for Detecting Bone Stress Injury**

	MRI	Bone Scintigraphy (BS)	Ultrasound (US)
Sensitivity	86–100%	74–84%	83%
Specificity	100%	33%	76%

relative energy deficiency in sport (RED-S) when evaluating and managing bone stress injury in the runner.

The syndrome of RED-S refers to physiologic impairment secondary to relative energy deficiency, or low energy availability (LEA). LEA occurs when the athlete's energy intake does not equal the energy expended during exercise. The result of this mismatch is inadequate energy supply to support and maintain health and performance. Signs of RED-S include gonadal dysfunction, weight loss, recurrent injury, disordered eating, mood changes, and more. The Female Athlete Triad (low bone mineral density, menstrual dysfunction, and disordered eating) is one component of RED-S. While LEA is difficult to measure objectively, a decent surrogate marker is BMI <17.5 kg/m^2, though this extreme is not a mandatory criterium for LEA. Athletes with low BMI are at increased risk for low bone mineral density in both sexes, which translates to increased risk for BSI.

If RED-S is suspected, it is important to get a multidisciplinary team involved early, including a sports dietician, sports psychologist, and potentially an endocrinologist. A physician experienced in the care of athletes could be the lead for this team of consultants, manage the musculoskeletal injury, and help with an appropriate plan for return to sport. The dietician can calculate current energy balance and initiate an appropriate dietary plan. The psychologist can evaluate for any mood disturbance as well as assist in the runner's adjustment to their disability (i.e. not being able to run). The endocrinologist can evaluate for causes other than standard hypothalamic amenorrhea as a source of low bone density, if in fact a bone densitometry (DXA) scan confirms low bone density (see Table 22.4). If there is concern for disordered eating or poor nutrition, especially in the case of bone stress injury, screening for Vitamin D deficiency is appropriate. Improving vitamin D deficiency may reduce healing time and facilitate earlier return to sport in cases of BSI.

The management of the runner with a BSI is generally described as a two-phase protocol. Phase one focuses on rest and pain control, while phase two focuses on progressive return to running. When the athlete stops running, the pain of a BSI usually dissipates quickly, and pain medication is often not needed. Nonsteroidal anti-inflammatory drugs (NSAIDs) should be avoided to limit the possible effect of impaired bone-healing.

TABLE 22.4 Indications for Bone Density Testing (DXA Scan) in Athletes

≥ 1 "High-Risk" Factors	≥ 2 "Moderate-Risk" Factors
Two prior BSI's, one high-risk BSI, or a low-energy nontraumatic fracture	One prior BSI
Prior Z-score of <–2.0 (after at least 1 year from baseline DXA)	Prior Z-score between –1.0 and –2.0 (after at least 1 year interval from baseline DXA)
BMI ≤17.5 kg/m², <85% estimated weight, or recent weight loss of ≥10% in 1 month	BMI between 17.4 and 18.5, <90% estimated weight, or recent weight loss of 5–10% in 1 month
Menarche ≥16 years of age	Menarche between ages 15 and 16 years
Current or history of <6 menses over 12 months	Current or history of 6–8 menses over 12 months
History of a DSM-5 diagnosed eating disorder	Current or history of disordered eating for 6 months or greater

Non-pharmacologic therapy to increase energy availability is the mainstay of treatment for the athlete with RED-S and BSI. Bisphosphonates are generally not indicated for low BMD or fracture reduction in premenopausal athletes. Long-term bisphosphonate use has been associated with atypical femur fractures, osteonecrosis, and teratogenicity. Bisphosphonates are rarely considered in an athlete with very low BMD and significant fracture history with lack of response to non-pharmacologic therapy. The use of combined oral contraceptives (COC) to regain menses or improve BMD is also not recommended. If menstrual cycles do not return after a reasonable trial of multidisciplinary interventions to improve energy availability, transdermal estradiol (E2) therapy with cyclic oral progestin can be considered for short-term use. The athlete should be counseled that this is not a reliable contraceptive method.

Guiding the runner in cross-training activities that can be implemented to maintain cardiovascular fitness is important and can typically start early once pain free. Cross-training can also facilitate an easier return to land running when ready. Two sport-specific modalities for cross-training the injured runner include deep water running and antigravity treadmill training. Deep water running simulates the biomechanics of running and has been shown to achieve a metabolic response comparable to running on land, while at the same time maintaining on-land running performance. Antigravity treadmill training involves a treadmill connected to an air-filled, pressure-controlled chamber that surrounds the lower half of the body and is able to unweight the body. Typically, athletes start training at 60–65% body weight and gradually increase the percentage as they remain pain free during and after training. Once the runner is able to tolerate 85–90% body weight, they can start to slowly introduce on-land running. If these modalities are not available, there are many progressive walk/jog programs that facilitate a gradual return to running, but these need to begin later when the fracture is further along in the healing process.

In general, the runner should be pain free with ambulation and cross-training for at least 2 weeks before returning to land-based running. They should begin on-land running at no more than half the usual distance and at a slower pace. They can then start gradually increasing distance, duration, and intensity. Intensity should only be increased once the runner has returned to typical distance and duration of training runs. In the case of a sacrum/pelvis BSI, which takes longer to heal then many other BSIs, general guidance is 7–12 weeks before returning to land running (clinical experience suggests this recommendation is closer to 12 weeks), remembering that any increase in activity should be pain free. Due to the prolonged healing of a sacral BSI, it is important to make the diagnosis early.

Physical therapy can be utilized to improve any mechanical deficiencies that may have contributed to the original injury, to perform video running gait analysis, and to facilitate the gradual return to the run plan. Referral to a sports medicine physician should be considered for the high-level athlete or an athlete with a time-sensitive goal who would benefit from more sport-specific rehabilitation to expedite recovery and return to sport.

1. Runners are prone to a number of specific injuries which may cause LBP including bone stress injuries.
2. It is crucial to collect a comprehensive medical and training history including prior running-related injuries and signs of potential relative energy deficiency in sport (RED-S).
3. Evaluation in clinic should involve a functional assessment including dynamic testing to uncover biomechanical deficits that are likely to be amplified when fatigue develops during training.
4. With a bone stress injury, it is not safe for the runner to continue to run until they have rested appropriately and completed an appropriate rehabilitation and a graded return to run program.
5. Cross-training the injured athlete should begin early, once they are pain free, in order to maintain cardiovascular fitness.

Further reading

1. De Souza MJ, Nattiv A, Joy E, et al. 2014 Female Athlete Triad Coalition consensus statement on treatment and return to play of the female athlete triad: 1st International Conference held in San Francisco, California, May 2012 and 2nd International Conference held in Indianapolis, Indiana, May 2013. Br J Sports Med. 2014;48:289.
2. Harrast MA. Clinical Care of the Runner: Assessment, Biomechanical Principles, and Injury Management. Elsevier, 2020.
3. Liem BC, Truswell HJ, Harrast MA. Rehabilitation and return to running after lower limb stress fractures. Curr Sports Med Rep. 2013;12(3):200–207.
4. Mountjoy M, Sundgot-Borgen J, Burke L, et al. International Olympic Committee (IOC) consensus statement on Relative Energy Deficiency in sport (RED-S): 2018 update. International Journal of Sport Nutrition and Exercise Metabolism. 2018;28(4):316–331.

23 "My Back Is OK as Long as I Don't Do Anything, but I Love Soccer and Tennis.": Back Pain in a Recreational Athlete

Maria A. Vanushkina, Christopher J. Standaert

A 45-year-old presents with intermittent low back pain. They report being extremely active, playing in an indoor tennis league in the winter and for 2 soccer teams in the spring and summer. They work as a paralegal, largely doing desk and computer-based work. Gyms, fitness classes, and similar things have never been appealing to them. Over the past 6 months, they have experienced low back pain frequently with soccer or tennis, which, on average, they participate in 4 or 5 days per week. The pain is not problematic with work or daily activities at home. Although a bit tight in the low back at times, your patient does not really stretch but does take over the counter nonsteroidal anti-inflammatories before playing soccer or tennis. They note their job is busy, and they tend to go directly to practice from work most of the time. There is no leg pain or neurologic change, and radiographs show some loss of disc height and small osteophytes at several levels in their lumbar spine.

What do you do now?

t is clear that sports are an important part of this patient's life and every effort should be made to support this patient in safely continuing both tennis and soccer for as long as they desire to do so. Reassurance and counseling is the most important component in managing this case.

Some patients may want to obtain an MRI at this stage. Obtaining further imaging without a trial of medical management would be nonconcordant with best practice guidelines. It is sometimes tempting to be more aggressive with both imaging and treatment in athletes than in the general population. Research and guidelines do not support this behavior. Risks associated with non-guideline imaging include unnecessary radiation exposure, increased rates of surgery, and patient labeling. The phenomenon of labeling has been shown to worsen patients' sense of well-being. In general, advanced imaging should be saved for patients for whom noninvasive, conservative regimens have failed, and therapeutic injection or surgery are being considered.

Many athletes will have questions about the effects of sports participation on LBP and structural damage to the spine. LBP is incredibly common across all demographics. However, LBP is less common in both elite athletes and regular exercisers than in the general population. Statistics help illustrate this point. By age 18, half of the pediatric population have experienced an episode of LBP. In any given year, up to 45% of adults will have an LBP episode, 2–8% will report one or more severe LBP episodes, and 8–13% experience chronic LBP (CLBP) lasting more than 3 months. The lifetime prevalence of LBP is up to 90% in the general population. The reported prevalence of LBP in competitive athletes is 1–40%, and the lifetime prevalence is only about 60%. The universal expert consensus is that exercise seems to be protective against LBP and has a multitude of other health benefits. The data on the effects of specific sports on structural changes in the spine are more limited and more controversial. There is some evidence that certain sports (not the two in this case) may increase the prevalence of degenerative findings on imaging, especially if single-sport participation without cross-training starts in childhood or adolescence; however, these degenerative findings appear to be minimally correlated with LBP episodes.

Our patient, like in most cases, is not reporting any specific injury that provoked their symptoms. In studies of LBP, the majority of episodes are unprovoked in onset or attributed to low energy "trauma," such as picking something up or making an awkward movement during an activity. Older athletes are more likely than the younger population to sustain musculoskeletal injuries during sports. Degenerative changes to the joints and tendons as well as muscular deconditioning and sarcopenia become factors that can contribute to higher injury rates as well as decreased performance and pain events in the aging population.

In an otherwise healthy adult without pain, starting in their 30s, metabolism will begin to slow noticeably enough to start adding fat to the body—about 2–3% every decade. Muscle mass loss will also begin, averaging 3–8% every decade. These changes will continue for life. In the fifth decade, additional changes begin to occur affecting the patient's cardiovascular system. Functionally, the maximum heart rate starts to drop, cardiac output decreases and VO2 max starts to decrease. Men in their 40s begin to have higher risks for cardiac disease. If not already doing so, it is important to start a combination of aerobic exercise and strength training to counteract these changes.

To compound the effects of aging on the body, episodes of pain may lead to periods of immobility and more rapid physical deconditioning. There are small but measurable amounts of muscle loss that occur due to immobility, around 0.5% loss per day, and possibly even faster loss in older patients. Back pain is associated with significant changes in physical performance measures, as well as neurologic changes in movements and recruitment patterns, shortening of muscles and connective tissue, and loss of Type 2 muscle fibers. Fortunately, most of those changes are reversible. A variety of therapeutic exercise programs result in meaningful improvements in range of motion, flexibility, strength, lifting capacity, and endurance. There is also evidence for reversal of changes associated with muscle atrophy from immobility for patients with subacute and chronic pain. Although skeletal muscles are thought of as having very limited regenerative properties, exercise is one of a few known interventions for promoting myogenesis (the formation of skeletal muscle).

In this case presentation, the patient needs to practice better self-care in order to reduce their pain symptoms now as well as to maintain their fitness and performance goals as they age. Relevant modifiable factors include a sedentary job, no current stretching or strength training program, and an expressed reluctance to participate in structured exercise regimens. The remainder of the visit should be spent on reviewing strategies on remedying these factors.

This patient, and most patients with LBP, should be advised to continue their work and recreational activities as tolerated, despite a pain episode. Alternative means of getting aerobic exercise to maintain overall conditioning should be reviewed if pain symptoms limit typical sports participation. In cases of mild symptoms, as with the presenting case, it is often safe to continue recreational sport participation without restrictions. Patients should avoid severely aggravating their symptoms beyond a 2/10 change on the pain scale. Patients with moderate or severe symptoms may benefit from a short period of relative rest from the sport until pain is more manageable. During this period of rest, patients should still be encouraged to stretch and move as much as they can.

Our specific patient could be encouraged to spend less time sitting at work and implement strategies to incorporate breaks for stretching throughout the workday. An ergonomic evaluation at work is unlikely to be of benefit, however, as there are no major symptoms during work. The importance of cross-training and strength training should be reinforced on multiple occasions. There are many ways to perform strength training without going to the gym or participating in organized classes. The patient's reasons and motivations for following through on this treatment recommendation should be elicited to help with goal setting and compliance. Additionally, a more detailed physical exam may be helpful to assess for trunk and limb range of motion deficits, as well as asymmetry or imbalances in strength during functional tasks like single-leg sit to stand. Sometimes having these changes pointed out serves as motivation for athletically minded patients, who may not otherwise be aware of these imbalances and their effect on sports performance.

A referral to physical therapy can be considered in this situation, although it may not be necessary with a self-motivated individual. If physical therapy is pursued, setting realistic expectations and goals as well as maintaining consistent education between the physician and physical therapist is helpful in optimizing outcomes. The treatment should focus on restoring trunk and limb range of motion and strength, building endurance, correcting biomechanical issues during sports-specific activities, and creating a sustainable home program for maintaining performance. Some patients may be interested in working with a sport-specific trainer or coach instead of a physical therapist. The evidence on efficacy of biomechanical correction alone is inconclusive on meta-analysis.

Many athletes may initially feel skeptical about the benefits of cross-training or physical therapy on top of their baseline activities. Data suggest that even elite athletes have dysfunctional movement patterns in their core stabilizers during episodes of LBP. The mainstay of treatment is exercise-based rehabilitation. In the general population, treatments that restore full trunk range of motion and full trunk strength and neuromuscular control have the best supporting evidence for reducing acute and chronic LBP symptoms. However, addressing physical impairments alone does not seem to be enough on its own to fully resolve pain and disability in every case of LBP. Nonetheless, studies consistently show that function and physical performance can be improved through exercise without worsening the pain experience.

Exercise also affects neuronal physiology as it pertains to pain. There is a phenomenon termed "exercise induced hypoalgesia." In animal studies of pain and injury, exercise reverses some of the injury-induced neurologic changes in sensory ganglia, spinal cord, and brain. The effects of exercise on pain appear to be generalized and not specific to the exercise performed. Pain appears to be reduced in exercising animals even if the exercise excludes the injured body part. Similar evidence is gradually accruing in humans as well. Patients may benefit from counseling regarding the potential temporary exacerbation of their symptoms when beginning a new exercise program. Fortunately, in the case of most spinal disorders without structural instability, it is safe to push through this pain as tolerated when exercising.

Medications and other modalities may be used to temporarily reduce pain and improve participation in rehabilitation efforts. Nonsteroidal anti-inflammatory drugs (NSAIDs) and thermal treatments have the highest level of evidence. This patient is taking NSAIDs four to five times per week to manage their symptoms, which appears to be an effective strategy. Given the known side effects associated with NSAIDs, this patient should be monitored for these periodically and renal function should be monitored biannually if the patient remains on this dose consistently. It may be beneficial to suggest topical heat or cold as an alternative or adjuvant pain relief option. Muscle relaxers have limited supporting evidence and are often too sedating to be used during the daytime. These are not appropriate for this case given no symptoms outside of sports. Spinal manipulation has low evidence for efficacy in acute symptoms, with a recent meta-analysis on the subject once again showing inconclusive results. More aggressive interventions such as spinal injections are not appropriate in this situation.

It is important to keep in mind that LBP is often an episodic condition. Once a patient has been successfully rehabilitated and returned to their desired sport participation, it is important to establish a maintenance plan. The patient in our case should be encouraged to continue both stretching and cross-training to combat age-related physiologic changes to their musculoskeletal system. Doing these two to three times per week appears to be adequate. Establishing a plan for self-care in the event of recurrent pain episodes is also helpful. If symptoms persist or recur despite appropriate care, shared decision-making should be used to determine if the benefits of ongoing tennis and soccer participation at current intensities outweigh the cost to the patient. If needed, helping the patient come up with alternative ways to engage in sports and exercise is valuable as is discussing realistic performance expectations. For some patients, lowering expectations of their own performance due to aging may be challenging mentally and may be a difficult adjustment that requires some time.

KEY POINTS

1. Sport participation does not typically increase the prevalence of LBP, with evidence suggesting that regular vigorous activity is actually protective against LBP.
2. Athletes should be treated following similar guidelines to the general population; avoid aggressive imaging and interventions as there are no data to support them.
3. Activity recommendations during the recovery phase are unique to the specific patient; as a general rule, activities as tolerated should be encouraged.
4. Encouraging self-care including strength training, stretching, and discussion of realistic performance expectations with aging is important.

5. Physical therapy is the most helpful modality for management of acute and chronic LBP in athletes and the general population.

Further reading

1. Daniels JM, Pontius G, El-Amin S, et al. Evaluation of low back pain in athletes. Sports Health. 2011;3(4):336–345.
2. Kamalapathy PN, Hassanzadeh H. Spinal care in the aging athlete. Clin Sports Med. 2021;40(3):571–584.
3. Stevans JM, Delitto A, Khoja SS, et al. Risk factors associated with transition from acute to chronic low back pain in US patients seeking primary care. JAMA Netw Open. 2021;4(2):e2037371.
4. Thornton JS, Caneiro JP, Hartvigsen J, et al. Treating low back pain in athletes: a systematic review with meta-analysis. Br J Sports Med. 2021;55(12):656–662.
5. Trumees E. Low back pain in the aging athlete. Semin Spine Surg. 2010;22(4):222–233.

24 "I Go on This Golf Trip Every Year, but It Hurts to Swing a Club.": Back Pain and Golf

Seth Bires, Christopher J. Standaert, Prakash Jayabalan

A long-established patient comes to see you about his back. He is 54 with hypertension, a BMI of 32, and dyslipidemia. He plays golf sporadically but has been noting some problems with his low back lately while playing. His back does not particularly bother him at work or home. He does not exercise much beyond home projects. Whenever he takes more than a few swings with a golf club, his low back hurts. There is no real radiation into the legs. He has been doing basic stretching and some sit-ups at home, but this does not seem to help. He has taken yearly golf trips with his childhood friends for decades. They typically play golf every day for 7 days. This year, he is worried that his back pain will get in the way. He plans to leave for his trip in 3 months.

What do you do now?

Golf is one of the most popular recreational sports in the United States, with 26 million people playing at least one round of golf per year. Along with being an enjoyable and often social activity for many, golfing is also considered a moderate level physical activity. Engaging in golf can be an important part of maintaining an appropriate level of exercise. For those who enjoy golf, addressing musculoskeletal issues that may limit their ability to play can be beneficial for their physical and mental health.

Low back pain (LBP) is one the most common injuries seen in golfers, both professionally and recreationally, accounting for 25% of all golf injuries. Multiple factors have been linked to the increased risk of LBP in golfers, including the repetitive nature of the golf swing, carrying a golf bag, and some individual demographics and physical characteristics. There are also multiple biomechanical and neuromuscular factors that have been proposed to contribute to the development of LBP in golfers. Being of older age and male sex have been shown to have a significant association with LBP in both professional and recreational golfers. Golfers with higher BMI also have an increased risk of developing LBP secondary to golf, thought to be related to increased lumbar spinal loading during the golf swing. Another strong predictor of developing LBP with golf is having a previous history of LBP. Our patient described above meets many of the demographic factors that would put him at a higher risk, most notably his gender, advancing age, and current BMI of 32, placing him in the obese category.

LBP in golfers is typically related to cumulative stresses from the repetitive nature of the golf swing, as opposed to isolated trauma. The golf swing can be performed more than 50 times during a single round or up to 300 times during a typical practice session. It is a complex motion using muscles and joints throughout almost the entire body, requiring coordination and muscle endurance. Over the last 60 years, there has also been an evolution of the golf swing to emphasize more power and clubhead speed to improve the distance a ball travels. This requires extensive trunk rotation and high velocities of movement, which can put considerable stress on the low back.

To help golfers with LBP, it is useful to understand the biomechanics of the golf swing (see Figure 24.1) Prior to a swing, golfers typically address the golf ball standing with their feet shoulder-width apart, knees flexed to 20–25 degrees, and trunk flexed to approximately 45 degrees. This stance allows the golfer to establish a stable foundation for their swing, centering

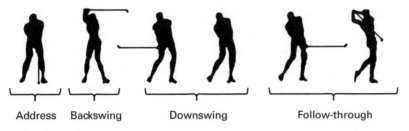

| Address | Backswing | Downswing | Follow-through |

FIGURE 24.1. Phases of the golf swing.

their weight over their feet. The lead foot (left foot for a right-handed swing, right foot for a left-handed swing) is angled somewhat toward the target to facilitate pelvic rotation and to reduce torsional loads on the spine during the backswing. The amount of lumbar flexion at address has been proposed as a contributor to LBP, with more flexion leading to greater stresses through the remainder of the swing.

The modern golf swing consists of three major phases. Phase 1, the backswing, begins when the clubhead moves back, away from the ball. This motion is achieved through activation of the trunk muscles (external and internal oblique and paraspinal muscles), rotating the clubhead and trunk away from the target. The pelvis and spine both rotate, but pelvic rotation is about half of thoracic rotation, adding torque to the torso and allowing for maximal energy production in the downswing. The difference between the rotation of the pelvis and rotation of the trunk is termed the "X-factor." A larger X-factor (greater disassociation of pelvic and trunk rotation) has been shown to increase stress on the lumbar spine. Many golfers will try to increase their X-factor in hopes of hitting the ball further.

Once the golfer has reached the top of their backswing, they will then initiate Phase 2, the downswing, by forcefully contracting the hip and knee extensors of the back leg. This coordinated firing causes the pelvis to slide laterally while the pelvis and trunk rotate toward the target. As the downswing progresses, the lead internal obliques and trail side external obliques fire to assist in accelerating trunk rotation. There is also increased side-bending toward the back leg which peaks along with trunk angular velocity at ball impact and during early follow-through. Greater amounts of lumbar side-bending toward the back leg may also increase the risk of injury.

Follow-through is the third and final phase of the golf swing. Following ball impact, the pelvis and trunk continue to rotate toward the target, concluding in a hyper-extended position of the spine with the trailing shoulder facing the target. During this phase, the spine experiences multiple cumulative forces, and it has been suggested that 41% of low back injuries are sustained around impact and during the early follow-through phase of the golf swing. To counteract these forces, the erector spinae and lead external obliques muscles continue to fire throughout the follow-through, likely playing an important role in decelerating the rotation of the trunk and maintaining low back stability. Poor endurance, strength, and coordination of these muscles may leave the golfer vulnerable to injury. Excessive lumbar rotation and extension during the follow-through phase can further increase stress throughout the lumbar spine.

With this understanding of the golf swing, we can work through a clinical approach to the golfer with LBP. Golfers are prone to the same issues that can affect all individuals, including disc problems, degenerative processes such as degenerative spondylolisthesis and spinal stenosis, and more concerning pathologies such as fractures, tumors, and infections. Specifically for the golfer, common causes of pain include muscle strains, inflammation or aggravation of underlying degenerative issues, and disc injuries. All of these can be related to the dynamics of the golf swing and the relative fitness, skill, flexibility, and motor control of the individual golfer. Because of the asymmetric nature of the golf swing, injuries typically occur more frequently on the side of the trail leg. As stated above, excessive flexion at the address phase, side-bending during the swing phase, and lumbar extension and over-rotation during the follow-through phase can all contribute to LBP (see Table 24.1). Proper muscle endurance, particularly of the abdominal, spine, and hip muscles, is critical in reducing cumulative stresses in the spine throughout the swing.

The history and examination of the golfer with LBP are intended to elicit deficits in training, knowledge, skill, or physical function that would predispose the golfer to problems with their lumbar spine. Specific to golfers, history should include previous LBP with golf, as well as the amount of general and golf-specific activity the patient performs on a regular basis. This can help assess the patient's baseline muscular endurance. In addition to the basic low back exam presented in earlier chapters, the

TABLE 24.1 **Common Problems in the Golf Swing that may be Associated with LBP**

Phases of Golf Swing	Common Biomechanical Problems
Pre-swing: Address	Excessive lumbar flexion
Phase 1: Backswing	Excessive trunk rotation in relationship to the amount of pelvic rotation (X-factor)
Phase 2: Downswing	Excessive side-bending toward the back leg
Phase 3: Follow-through	Excessive lumbar rotation and extension

physical exam for a golfer should include range of motion and strength testing of hips, as well as dynamic testing of hip and core stability. This can be achieved through single-leg stance and single-leg squats for assessing hip control.

In general, the literature has shown exercise to be the most effective method of treating pain and increasing function in those with LBP. In addition, it is relatively safe and provides many other important health benefits. Given the complex movement patterns required for a golf swing, it is important to correct golf-specific asymmetry and restrictions in lumbar and/ or hip range of motion and to improve the endurance of the trunk and hip musculature in golfers.

For the patient presented here, it would be most helpful to refer them for physical therapy. Initially, he should abstain from golf while any asymmetries or balance or strength deficits are addressed with safe, gradual progression back to golfing. During this period, he should be encouraged to engage in at least 30 minutes of moderate intensity aerobic exercise (walking or cycling for example) five times per week. The physical therapy program should focus on static postural strength, stability, balance, and range of motion with gradual functional progression toward golf-specific movements. This approach will also allow him to develop appropriate muscular endurance and minimize the potential for reinjury. As his BMI is 32, weight loss should be recommended, potentially with the assistance of a dietician. Explaining that poor fitness and excess weight may be related to his LBP which is, in turn, affecting his ability to play golf may provide added motivation.

Further medical workup is not necessarily required for this patient. Plain radiographs with standing antero/posterior, neutral lateral, and flexion/extension films may be helpful in assessing for scoliosis, a spondylolisthesis or other bony issues that could potentially influence physical therapy. If his examination shows significantly restricted hip range or motion or pain with hip exam, radiographs of the hips would be appropriate. Obtaining an MRI for this patient, in the absence of radicular pain or neurological issues, may be counterproductive. Given his age, it is highly likely he will have some degree of degenerative change on imaging (see chapter 4). It is also highly *unlikely* that any age-related degenerative changes are specifically causative of his pain. His treatment needs to focus on fitness, flexibility, neuromuscular control, endurance, and proper training for his sport. Medicalizing what are normal, expected findings for his age may lessen his confidence in his spine and lead him away from the fundamental need to address appropriate rehabilitation and training. There are no indications for spinal injections or surgical referral. Nonsteroidal anti-inflammatory drugs could be considered for short-term relief or pain, if necessary, but the primary treatment here will be a combination of physical therapy and exercise.

Although there are no current guidelines for safe return to golf after a low back injury, it is important that patients gradually increase repetitions while focusing on improving the biomechanics of the swing that limit stress on the low back. Referring the patient to a certified golf instructor may be beneficial to improving posture and biomechanics. A useful resource for the player is the Titleist Performance Institute (TPI) which provides online resources for golf-specific drills and exercise. They also provide certification in golf assessments from musculoskeletal practitioners including physical therapists (a directory of certified practitioners is available on their website). Once the patient does return to the golf course, it would be advisable to recommend that they walk the course as opposed to riding in a golf cart to optimize the health benefits of the sport. As carrying a golf bag has also been shown to put asymmetric loads through the lumbar spine, a wheeled golf push-cart may be advisable. Given that this patient's trip is 3 months away, it is realistic that he will be able to safely participate in his yearly golf trip after activity modification, physical therapy, and general functional progression back into golf.

1. Golf is a popular recreational activity that provides both physical and mental health benefits.
2. LBP is one of the most common injuries seen in golfers, accounting for 25% of all golf injuries in both professional and amateur golfers.
3. Male sex, advanced age, history of LBP, and increased BMI have been linked with the development of LBP in golfers.
4. Examination of golfers should include a thorough physical exam assessing range of motion of the lumbar spine, pelvis (rotation), and hips and testing of functional hip and abdominal strength.
5. Physical therapy and regular exercise are the primary initial treatments for LBP in golfers, concentrating on flexibility, core strength, endurance, and eventually golf swing mechanics.
6. When medically appropriate, golfers should be encouraged to walk the golf course due to the inherent health benefits of walking over using a golf cart.

Further reading
1. Murray AD, Daines L, Archibald D, et al. The relationships between golf and health: a scoping review. Br J Sports Med. 2017;51:12–19.
2. Smith JA. Hawkins A, Grant-Beuttler M, Beuttler R, Lee S-P. Risk factors associated with low back pain in golfers: a systematic review and meta-analysis. Sports Health. 2018;10(6):538–546.
3. Cole MH, Grimshaw PN. The biomechanics of the modern golf swing: implications for lower back injuries. Sports Med. 2016 Mar;46(3):339–351. doi: 10.1007/s40279-015-0429-1. PMID: 26604102.
4. Lindsay DM, Vandervoort AA. Golf-related low back pain: a review of causative factors and prevention strategies. Asian J Sports Med. 2014;5(4):e24289.
5. Patel ND, Broderick DF, Burns J, et al. ACR appropriateness criteria low back pain. J Am Coll Radiol. 2016;13(9):1069–1078.

25 "It Hurt So Much I Had to Come out of the Game.": A 14-Year-Old Soccer Player with Acute Low Back Pain

Kuntal Chowdhary, Christopher J. Standaert

A 14-year-old comes to see you for relatively acute low back pain. They are an avid soccer player, playing year-round for the last 5 years. This past year, they started high school and played for their high school team in the spring. They added this training onto the work with their established club/travel team. Near the end of high school season, they developed left-sided low back pain. This came on over a few days and progressed rapidly in severity. They had to stop playing and practicing about 3 weeks ago. The pain has gone down with resting at home, but it flared with just trying to run and do some drills in practice a few days ago. They have no leg pain. It hurts to flex or extend their spine. They have a soccer camp scheduled for next month, and their fall club season starts shortly after that. They are in your office with both parents today who want to know what is wrong and what to do about camp next month.

What do you do now?

Low back pain (LBP) is a surprisingly common complaint seen in children and adolescents in pediatric clinics. Unfortunately, the prevalence of axial LBP in children and adolescents and subsequent office visits have steadily been increasing over the past several years. In fact, the prevalence of LBP by age 18 approaches lifetime prevalence rates of LBP documented in adults, nearing 20% yearly prevalence and 75% lifetime prevalence. Accordingly, an estimated 24% of all adolescents seek medical attention for LBP, presenting a considerable health care burden. Despite numerical similarities to adults, however, the etiologies and evaluation of LBP are different in adolescents than in adults. Adolescents are more prone to bone rather than disc injuries, and there tend to be higher concerns for spinal deformities, inflammatory processes, and neoplasm. Importantly for this case, adolescent athletes represent a distinct population in considering LBP. The most common cause of LBP in an adolescent athlete who seeks medical attention and cannot play their sport is a fracture of the pars interarticularis of the neural arch of the vertebra, otherwise termed "isthmic spondylolysis."

When considering adolescents in general, there are several risk factors that can predispose given individuals to LBP. Non-modifiable risk factors include female sex, prior low back injury, family history of LBP, age, and ethnicity (with a higher prevalence in Black followed by White people, Hispanics, and American Indian/Alaskan Native). Modifiable risk factors include childhood obesity, sports specialization during adolescence, level of competition, and other psychosocial and socioeconomic factors. The psychosocial environment of an adolescent can have profound effects on their health, in general, and influence complaints of pain. Poverty, trauma, abuse, anxiety, depression, isolation, school or social stress, bias, discrimination, fear or distrust of the health care system, and other psychosocial factors may affect adolescents in ways that are distinct from adults. Caring for these patients requires attention to their psychological state, their home, school, and social environments, and their developmental status. Autonomy and the influence of parents or caregivers on the history and physical exam need to be considered as well.

As with adults, it is frequently difficult to ascertain a clear structural cause for many adolescents with LBP, and providers need to be aware of the complexities of a given adolescent's psychosocial state. Disc herniations can occur in adolescents but are far less frequent than in the adult population.

Scoliosis of greater than 10° occurs in about 2% of adolescents (about 4% of females and less than 1% of males) but rarely presents with pain. Scheuermann's disease (hyper-kyphosis of the thoracic spine) with endplate irregularities and Schmorl's nodes can be painful in adolescents, manifesting with a dull, achy pain typically at the thoracolumbar junction. Other bone injuries may occur, such as a fracture of the ring apophysis of the vertebral body. Adolescents also may present with inflammatory conditions, such as spondyloarthropathies like ankylosing spondylitis (see chapter 30) or juvenile idiopathic arthritis. Young individuals are also at risk for tumors, which may be benign or malignant in nature, and infections, including discitis, vertebral osteomyelitis, and epidural abscess. These three conditions may also be associated with fever, which is not typical of the other etiologies described above.

In adolescent athletes presenting with LBP, isthmic spondylolysis is far and away the most common cause of pain identified. This should be considered the diagnosis of exclusion in almost any adolescent athlete who self-limits sports participation due to LBP, and all of these individuals warrant appropriate diagnostic evaluation. In tracing the etymology of the words from Greek, "spondyl" means "vertebra," "-lysis" means "loosening," and "-olisthesis" means "to slip." Given this, "spondylolysis" refers to a separation or fracture of the vertebral arch while "spondylolisthesis" refers to an actual slip or forward translation of one vertebral body over the one below it. Although similar in origins and name, the fracture (spondylolysis) and slip (spondylolisthesis) are different conditions. Not everyone with spondylolysis develops a spondylolisthesis, and there are causes of spondylolisthesis that are unrelated to spondylolysis (most particularly a degenerative spondylolisthesis, see chapter 9). Isthmic spondylolysis is a specific condition in which the fracture occurs in the pars interarticularis of the neural arch (see Figure 25.1). This is often simply termed "a pars fracture."

In studies of the general population, pars fractures are identified on plain radiographs in about 5% of individuals by age 6. Essentially all of the children in these studies were asymptomatic, and most remained so over the course of their lifetime. The prevalence of pars fractures does not change throughout adulthood, indicating that acute pars fractures are a very rare event in adults. Pars fractures are found more frequently in males than in

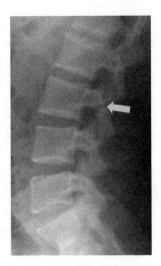

FIGURE 25.1. Plain radiograph of a 17-year-old with acute low back pain showing pars fractures/spondylolysis at L2 (arrow). There is no associated spondylolisthesis.

females. The rate is similar in Caucasians and those of Asian descent, lower for African Americans, and remarkably higher for the Inuit population. There is a strong association between isthmic spondylosis and congenital anomalies, such as spina bifida occulta. It is critically important to recognize that about 5% of asymptomatic adults and adolescents will have a pars fracture/spondylolysis on plain radiographs (see chapter 8). As these are not associated with pain, simply finding spondylolysis on radiographs does not help in diagnosing or treating LBP, either in the general population or adolescent athletes.

Adolescent athletes have an even higher background prevalence of pars fractures than does the population as a whole. In studies of elite adolescent athletes, the prevalence of spondylolysis on plain radiographs is approximately 8–15%, much higher than in the general population, with a male to female ratio of 2–3:1. It most commonly occurs in adolescent athletes involved in a sport that requires repetitive lumbar loading, notably extension and/or rotation. Spondylolysis is particularly frequent in weightlifters, wrestlers, throwing track and field athletes, divers, rowers, gymnasts, and soccer and tennis players. The theorized mechanism of action is associated with overuse with repetitive lumbar loading, especially hyperextension and rotary forces that lead to a fatigue fracture in the weakest part of the posterior vertebral arch, which is the pars interarticularis.

Adolescents with a painful pars lesion will describe LBP that can be diffuse or localized, typically centered in the L5 region, which is the most commonly affected lumbar level. The onset can be acute due to a traumatic or sentinel event or insidious in nature. The pain is typically relieved with rest and exacerbated with activity. It can be provoked by either flexion or extension of the spine, and there is no pathognomonic pattern of exacerbation and remission noted beyond relief with rest. Athletes frequently present with a pars injury following a rapid increase in training intensity (transitioning to high school or college sports, for example) or following a period of rapid growth. Typically, there is no radiation of the pain beyond the buttocks. True radicular/nerve root pain extending down the leg or the presence of neurologic complaints or findings in the leg would imply involvement of a nerve root and raise concern for either an associated spondylolisthesis or, less commonly, a disc herniation. In going through a patient's history, "red flag" symptoms must always be assessed, including severe pain (particularly at night), fevers, motor or sensory deficits, saddle anesthesia, and loss of bowel or bladder function.

Physical examination of the adolescent athlete incorporates some specific considerations given the unique circumstances of this age. For adolescents such as the one in the case above, inspection should include evaluation for any deformities (spondylolisthesis, scoliosis, or excessive thoracic kyphosis suggestive of Scheuermann's disease), rashes (association with inflammatory spondyloarthropathy), and hair tufts (spina bifida). A gait evaluation should be conducted, with particular attention to leg length discrepancy or pelvic obliquity, which may indicate a spinal deformity. Range of motion should be assessed, particularly flexion and extension within tolerance. For those with scoliosis, it is also useful to assess lateral flexion to assess for restriction of movement on the side of the curvature. In isthmic spondylolysis, the patient may experience pain to palpation over the affected bony area and possibly around the surrounding paraspinal musculature. As 85% of pars fractures and slips occur at L5/S1, neurologic exam needs to include muscles typically innervated by the L5 root such as tibialis anterior (ankle dorsiflexion), extensor hallucis longus (great toe extension), and gluteus medius (hip abduction). The neurologic exam is typically nonrevealing in patients with isthmic spondylolysis unless there is a concurrent spondylolisthesis with nerve root involvement.

The diagnosis of symptomatic isthmic spondylolysis requires diagnostic imaging. Given the high prevalence rates for asymptomatic pars fractures in the athletic population, simply identifying a pars fracture on plain radiograph is not diagnostic. Plain radiographs can generally be limited to standing anterior/posterior and flexion/extension views. Nuclear imaging (bone scan with single photon emission computed tomography (SPECT)), computed tomography (CT), and magnetic resonance imaging (MRI) are all considerations for further imaging. Choices here can be controversial. Bone scan with SPECT has clearly been shown to have the most utility in identifying a symptomatic pars lesion (see Figure 25.2). If this study is negative, it is highly unlikely the patient has a painful pars lesion. A positive SPECT study needs to be followed by a limited CT of the area of concern to clarify the nature of the bone lesion (osteoid osteomas, fractures in areas other than the pars, and other bone issues can result in a positive SPECT) and to stage the fracture for treatment stratification (see Figure 25.3). MRI is often used and has advantages as there is no associated ionizing radiation, and soft tissue pathology can be readily identified. However, MRI is less sensitive than SPECT/CT, missing approximately 20% of pars lesions,

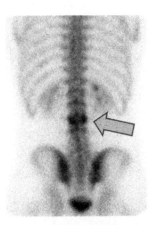

FIGURE 25.2. Planar bone scan of the same patient showing increased uptake bilaterally at L2 (arrow).

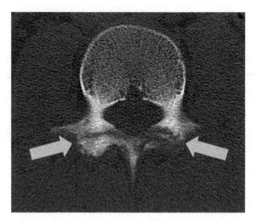

FIGURE 25.3. Axial CT scan of the same patient showing early-stage bilateral pars fractures (arrows).

and the false positive rate is unknown. Suspicion of a pars fracture on MRI should also prompt a CT to stage the lesion.

The natural history of spondylolysis is generally favorable clinically, with about 85% of athletes returning to play, but only about 30% of individuals actually heal their fractures. Healing rates vary by the type of fracture, and bilateral fractures that do not heal can develop a spondylolisthesis while those that heal their fractures essentially resolve the injury and will not develop a spondylolisthesis. Unilateral, early stage fractures heal at a very high rate, roughly 80% or more. Bilateral fractures have an overall healing rate of only about 20%, but those rates are higher for early stage lesions (see Figure 25.2). What are termed "terminal stage lesions" are essentially non-unions of bone with significant separation of the fracture and cortication of the bone. These do not heal. Treatment can be tailored to the likelihood of healing. Adequate rest to obtain healing of a unilateral early stage lesion has a high likelihood of resolving the injury. The bone heals, and the fracture is gone. The minimum time to healing is 3 months, with some fractures taking 4–6 months to heal. Athletes with these fractures should therefore limit stress to their spines (and sports activity) for at least 3 months. Those with terminal stage lesions just need to rest until symptom resolution as they will not heal.

Initial management of isthmic spondylolysis consists primarily of activity restriction (rest). Acute, early stage fractures need time to heal, so patients are advised to cease sports participation and only perform routine daily activities for 3 months, allowing for gradual resolution of pain. Additional exercise and physical therapy in this time frame are best avoided. Pain control can be managed with acetaminophen or nonsteroidal anti-inflammatory drugs (NSAIDs). Assuming rest results in the resolution of pain, after 3 months, a physical therapy regimen can be initiated, focusing on reconditioning, strengthening of the paraspinal and core musculature, and gradual progression through sports-specific training. Although there is no consensus on the specific physical therapy regimens that should be done, a few studies have shown that stretching of tight hamstring muscles and correction of lumbar lordosis are important, as both of these factors may contribute to isthmic spondylolysis. The use of lumbar bracing is controversial in the literature as clinical outcomes are equivalent with or without bracing. There is no evidence to support the routine use of bracing, and this is best avoided. Return to play is typically 6–7 months after the injury was diagnosed, implying that rehabilitation takes 3–4 months. If athletes do well with the above approach, there is no need for further imaging unless bilateral fractures are identified. In these patients, annual radiographs are needed during the adolescent growth spurt to monitor for progressive slip. There is no contraindication to play for a small slip, but larger or progressive slips warrant surgical consultation. If LBP is persistent and the fracture is not healing or a slip is progressing, surgical options can be considered. The most common surgical interventions are direct repair of the pars interarticularis defect or fusion of the lumbar segment to avoid progressive spondylolisthesis.

The patient presented here has a high probability of having a pars fracture and should be approached as described above. They should first be evaluated with limited plain radiographs but will need advanced imaging, as well. A bone scan with SPECT followed by a CT is the most sensitive combination of tests to identify and stage a symptomatic pars lesion. Given the radiation exposure associated with SPECT, MRI can be considered with the caveat that approximately 20% of pars interarticularis fractures are missed. If indicative of a fracture, the MRI should also be followed by a CT. The mainstay of treatment for symptomatic isthmic spondylolysis is an extended period of rest of approximately three months. Consideration should be given on whether the fracture is unilateral or bilateral, as bilateral fractures tend to not heal as well, and patients may require a more prolonged period of activity restriction. Following appropriate rest and after achieving full, pain-free range of lumbar motion, a physical therapy regimen can be initiated. However, caution should be given to take a gradual approach and not initiate physical therapy early in the course of healing, as this can result in recurrent pain and prolonged healing time. Therapy needs to start with an early focus on cardiovascular reconditioning, range of motion, and trunk stability and then steadily progress through sports-specific training, generally over a period of 3-4 months.

KEY POINTS

1. Approximately 5% of asymptomatic adults and adolescents and 10% of high level athletes will have a pars fracture/spondylolysis on plain radiographs.
2. Diagnosis of isthmic spondylolysis relies on advanced radiographic imaging to identify the presence of an acute/symptomatic pars lesion. Bone scan with SPECT followed by a CT of the lumbar spine is the most sensitive imaging approach.
3. The mainstay of treatment is a prolonged period of rest and activity restriction for at least 3 months.
4. Following the rest period, physical therapy should be initiated. The initial focus is on reconditioning and strengthening of the paraspinal and core musculature followed by a gradual transition through sport-specific training.
5. Return to play for an acute pars injury/spondylolysis is typically 6–7 months after diagnosis.

Further reading
1. Beutler WJ, Fredrickson BE, Murtland A, Sweeney CA, Grant WD, Baker D. The natural history of spondylolysis and spondylolisthesis: 45-year follow-up evaluation. Spine (Phila Pa 1976). 2003 May 15;28(10):1027–1035; discussion 1035. doi: 10.1097/01.BRS.0000061992.98108.A0. PMID: 12768144.
2. Klein G, Mehlman CT, McCarty M. Nonoperative treatment of spondylolysis and grade I spondylolisthesis in children and young adults: a meta-analysis of

observational studies. J Pediatr Orthop. 2009 Mar;29(2):146–156. doi: 10.1097/
BPO.0b013e3181977fc5. PMID: 19352240.

3. Masci L, Pike J, Malara F, Phillips B, Bennell K, Brukner P. Use of the one-legged
   hyperextension test and magnetic resonance imaging in the diagnosis of active
   spondylolysis. Br J Sports Med. 2006 Nov;40(11):940–946; discussion 946.
   doi: 10.1136/bjsm.2006.030023. Epub 2006 Sep 15. PMID: 16980534; PMCID:
   PMC2465027.

4. Standaert CJ, Herring SA. Expert opinion and controversies in sports and
   musculoskeletal medicine: the diagnosis and treatment of spondylolysis in
   adolescent athletes. Arch Phys Med Rehabil. 2007 Apr;88(4):537–540. doi: 10.1016/
   j.apmr.2007.01.007. PMID: 17398258.

5. Standaert CJ, Herring SA. Spondylolysis: a critical review. Br J Sports Med.
   2000 Dec;34(6):415–422. doi: 10.1136/bjsm.34.6.415. PMID: 11131228; PMCID:
   PMC1724260.

26 "My Injury Was Years Ago, but Something in My Back Is Not Right.": Low Back Pain on the Way to the Paralympics

Deborah Crane

Your 34-year-old patient sustained a T10 fracture with a spinal cord injury in a motor vehicle accident at age 20. They have no motor or sensory function below the T8 level and have used a manual wheelchair for ambulation ever since. About 3 years after the injury, your patient began playing wheelchair basketball. This has been a passion for your patient ever since. A driven individual, they excelled in the sport and have applied for a slot on the US National Team, hoping to play in the upcoming Paralympics. Although having no other significant health issues, your patient began having back pain about 3 months ago. It has become progressively worse. The pain clearly is exacerbated by playing basketball, but now anything beyond routine indoor ambulation with the wheelchair results in pain. The patient presents to your clinic asking what could be wrong and if there is something you can do to help them keep playing.

What do you do now?

Back pain in individuals with spinal cord injury (SCI) is common, and the few studies that have been done suggest that the majority of patients with SCI (estimates range from 50–83%) have low back pain (LBP) and/or trunk pain. For patients with SCI, back pain may be due to centrally mediated neuropathic pain arising from the injured spinal cord or may be pain related to poor mechanics with altered strength, seating issues, posttraumatic spine deformities, charcot spine, all structural in nature. Differentiating between these two types of pain is important in determining the cause and potential remedy for the patient's pain. Neuropathic pain tends to be described as burning, stabbing, or aching and generally occurs at the level of the SCI or below. Patients with thoracic-level SCI often describe a band-like or ring-like pain around their trunk at the level of their SCI. Typically, neuropathic pain does not present with specific exacerbating factors. In contrast, pain from a variety of spinal structures (e.g. bone, disc, ligament, muscle, etc.) is more commonly described as dull or achy and usually occurs above the level of injury. Movement or activity involving the affected structure or region tends to aggravate this type of pain.

SCI poses unique challenges in the clinical approach to LBP. Those with SCI may experience back pain as a result of muscular weakness and imbalance as well as altered biomechanics that result from these changes. Due to denervation of truncal musculature, many individuals have poor or altered posture. Lower extremity and trunk spasticity can contribute to LBP and difficulties maintaining posture. Conventional treatments for managing LBP such as core strengthening and lumbar stabilization exercises can be limited by the neuromuscular weakness or paralysis that results from SCI. Additionally, basic modalities commonly used to treat LBP, such as heat and ice, can be harmful and should be used with great caution in the SCI population due to risk of burns or other thermal injuries in the setting of impaired sensation.

Individuals with SCI with prior spinal trauma and surgical instrumentation are at risk of developing post-traumatic spinal deformities that may or may not be associated with pain. Post-traumatic kyphotic deformity is the most common of these, often due to compression fractures or complications of spinal instrumentation. Neuromuscular scoliosis is another possible deformity and occurs due to truncal muscle strength asymmetries. Increased kyphosis and scoliosis have been commonly thought to lead to pain.

However, studies have not particularly supported this theory, and questions remain about how much pain is associated with post-traumatic spinal deformities for patients with SCI.

Other possible causes of new onset back pain in individuals with SCI include hardware failure, post-traumatic syringomyelia, infection, fracture, and disc herniation. Many individuals with spinal trauma and SCI have undergone spinal instrumentation to stabilize fractures. Over time, there is risk of spinal instrumentation loosening, fracturing, or becoming infected. All of these scenarios could lead to new onset LBP in a patient with chronic SCI. New onset neuropathic pain that develops in a patient with SCI may be due to post-traumatic syringomyelia. In this condition, a syrinx, or fluid-filled cavity, forms in the spinal cord, often at the site of the initial injury. This can be associated with a change in the individual's neurological level as evidenced by an ascending loss of sensation or strength. Those with SCI may also be prone to developing compression fractures, and, like all individuals, can develop degenerative conditions or a disc herniation. These may present atypically in individuals with SCI due to baseline strength and sensory deficits as well as the frequent presence of baseline neuropathic pain and paresthesia below the level of injury.

One specific condition unique to individuals with impaired sensation in spinal segments, such as SCI, is neuropathic spinal arthropathy, or Charcot spine. Charcot spine tends to occur more in individuals with neurologically complete SCI resulting in a higher degree of paralysis and sensory loss below the injury level. The lack of normal protective sensory mechanisms allows for abnormal movement between vertebrae with destruction of bony surfaces, subchondral bone fractures, and vertebral collapse resulting in a pseudoarthrosis with frank instability (see Figure 26.1). Charcot spine is most common in the lumbar spine, below the level of original injury. LBP experienced in an otherwise insensate area is a hallmark presenting symptom. Spinal deformity (particularly increased kyphosis), crepitus (frequently described as an audible "grinding" or "clunking"), changes in spasticity and/or neurological function below the level of injury, symptoms of cauda equina compression, and loss of deep tendon reflexes can all occur with a Charcot spine. Patients with SCI at the level of T6 or above may also experience autonomic dysreflexia, a potentially life-threatening condition

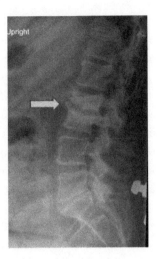

FIGURE 26.1.   Lateral radiograph of the lumbar spine radiograph showing L2/L3 disc and vertebral body destruction with sclerosis (arrow) consistent with the diagnosis of Charcot spine. These findings could also be seen with infection (discitis/osteomyelitis, see chapter 15).

where pain or discomfort below one's level of SCI results in autonomic instability and critical hypertension.

Plain radiographs of the thoracic and lumbar spine, ideally with flexion/ extension views, are essential to obtain in patients with SCI and new onset, impairing, or persisting LBP. These can identify hardware issues, spondylolisthesis, Charcot spine, and any progressive spinal deformity. Magnetic resonance imaging (MRI) of the lumbar spine is generally necessary to identify associated neurologic or spinal canal involvement, a disc herniation, syrinx, or infection. When assessing for a possible syrinx, imaging of the spinal cord with a thoracic or cervical MRI is required. When infection is a concern, MRI should be performed with and without intravenous (IV) contrast and laboratory studies (specifically an erythrocyte sedimentation rate (ESR), C-reactive protein (CRP), and white blood cell count (WBC)) should also be obtained (see chapter 15). Computed tomography (CT) may be necessary if bone detail on MRI is obscured by the presence of spinal instrumentation.

For all individuals with SCI using a wheelchair for mobility, ensuring optimal wheelchair positioning by a trained wheelchair seating specialist is essential to try to minimize musculoskeletal pain. An optimal wheelchair seat position and backrest will promote sitting stability and minimize unnecessary restrictions of truncal mobility. Stabilizing features can include an angled seat with the front of the seat higher than the rear. Low backrest height will reduce unneeded limitations in truncal mobility. The rear wheel axel should also be positioned two inches in front of the shoulder to minimize upper limb stress. Some studies have found that the vibrations experienced during daily activities by wheelchair users may exceed safety standards set by the trucking industry. It is difficult to mitigate this, but ensuring that the patient has an appropriately supportive and pressure-relieving wheelchair cushion can potentially reduce the risk of back pain due to vibration.

The patient presented in this case has a chronic T8 complete SCI resulting from a T10 fracture 14 years ago. The vignette describes new onset, worsening, back pain that is exacerbated with activity. This is more consistent with structural pain rather than neuropathic pain. Given the chronicity of the SCI, the presence of a neurologically complete injury, and location of a lower thoracic spinal fracture, the patient is at risk for Charcot spine. One should inquire about additional symptoms including crepitus or changes in neurological function, spasticity, or bowel and bladder function. This vignette indicates that the patient is not having any other significant health issues, but one will still want to inquire about systemic symptoms such as fever, chills, night sweats, and weight loss that could be consistent with infection or malignancy. Since the patient's SCI is at the T8 level (below the level of T6), it is unlikely that they would experience autonomic dysreflexia.

Physical examination should begin with inspection of the patient's posture in the wheelchair to help identify any spinal deformities such as kyphosis or scoliosis. One should palpate the spine for step-offs indicating frank instability. The location of the pain may be somewhat vague due to the patient's baseline sensory impairment. Neurologic examination should be performed to evaluate for changes in baseline sensory level, alterations in deep tendon reflexes (DTRs) and spasticity, and rectal tone or sensation. If a Charcot lesion results in compression of the spinal cord below the level of injury (potentially at or above L1), spasticity, DTRs, and rectal tone may increase. If the Charcot lesion affects the cauda equina (typically at or below L1), all of these may be reduced from baseline.

Given the physical exam limitations for a patient with sensory and motor deficits, this patient's presentation will warrant radiographs of their thoracic and lumbar spine with flexion and extension views. Comparing these to prior radiographs, if available, is helpful in detecting changes over time. In the case of Charcot spine, radiographs will reveal increasingly severe degenerative changes, bony destruction, and potential focal deformity (see Figure 26.1). CT can help to further evaluate osseous changes (see Figure 26.2) To differentiate Charcot spine from an infectious etiology, such as osteomyelitis, MRI with and without IV contrast, ESR, CRP, and WBC count will be helpful.

Charcot spine often requires surgical intervention. Once the diagnosis of Charcot spine is made, referral to neurosurgical or orthopedic spine specialists is essential. Surgical management of this condition typically requires extension of the spinal fusion with combined anterior and posterior fixation. Spinal immobilization with a thoracolumbosacral orthosis (TLSO) may be recommended as well. Unfortunately, recurrence

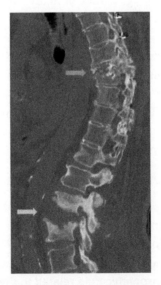

FIGURE 26.2. CT lateral reconstruction showing erosion/destruction of L2 and L3 with gapping at the L2/L3 disc space consistent with a diagnosis of Charcot spine (light arrow). This process is occurring below this individual's T6 injury level due to prior trauma to the mid-thoracic spine (darker arrow).

of Charcot spine is common. Providers caring for patients with a history of Charcot spine should maintain a high level of suspicion for recurrence and regularly monitor patients, inquiring about LBP and assessing for any changes in neurologic function or spasticity. Annual plain radiographs of the lumbar or thoracic spine may also be helpful.

It is thought that increasing upper trunk mobility, particularly in lateral bending and rotation, may increase destructive forces on the lower spine. For the patient in this case, their avid participation in wheelchair basketball at an elite level may be contributing to the development of a neuropathic joint. Unfortunately, it may be necessary to reduce participation in this and other recreational activities. This patient may then benefit from working with both a rehabilitation psychologist and a recreational therapist to help with alternative adaptive activities.

In the United States, SCI shows a strong male predominance and, historically, has been more common in younger individuals. With the aging of the US population, SCI has been seen in a bimodal distribution with males between 20–29 years old and over 70 years old being most at-risk. Over the last 50 years, the average age at time of injury has risen to 43 years. Most recent figures show that a higher proportion of SCI occurs in non-Hispanic Black people (24%) than are represented in the general population (13%). Research has shown that Black Americans with SCI report experiencing more discrimination and perceive greater racism in health care, along with higher levels of health care system distrust and lower health literacy than White people with SCI. As a result, Black people may be less likely to seek treatment when new symptoms arise and may have a delay in diagnosis and treatment for conditions like Charcot spine.

KEY POINTS

1. LBP is common in individuals with SCI, and the loss of sensory and motor function and potential trauma to the spinal column create unique diagnostic and treatment considerations.
2. Both ongoing neuropathic pain related to the primary SCI and post-traumatic spinal deformity affect many individuals with SCI.

3. New onset LBP should prompt consideration of structural injuries to the spinal cord (such as syringomyelia) or spinal column (such as a disc herniation, fracture, infection, hardware problem, or degenerative process).
4. As the ability of an individual with SCI to perceive pain below their level of injury may be altered and their neurological deficits may limit physical examination, it is critical to evaluate for any changes in neurological level of injury, spasticity/tone, and rectal tone as part of the routine evaluation for new onset LBP. There is also a greater reliance on the use of diagnostic imaging and laboratory studies than may be necessary in the non-SCI population.
5. Charcot spine is a relatively unique condition occurring below the level of injury in an individual with SCI and requires diagnostic imaging and surgical consultation/evaluation.

Further reading
1. Boninger, M, Saur, T, Trefler, E, Hobson, D, Burdett, R, Cooper, R. Postural changes with aging in tetraplegia: effects on life satisfaction and pain. Arch Phys Med Rehabil. 1998;79(12):1577–1581.
2. Goldstein B. Musculoskeletal conditions after spinal cord injury. Phys Med Rehabil Clin N Am. 2000 Feb;11(1):91–108, viii-ix. PMID: 10680160.
3. Miró J, Gertz KJ, Carter GT, Jensen MP. Pain location and functioning in persons with spinal cord injury. PM R. 2014 Aug;6(8):690–697. doi: 10.1016/j.pmrj.2014.01.010. Epub 2014 Jan 18. PMID: 24448429; PMCID: PMC4467570.
4. Solinsky R, Donovan JM, Kirshblum SC. Charcot Spine following chronic spinal cord injury: an analysis of 201 published cases. Spinal Cord. 2019 Feb;57(2):85–90. doi: 10.1038/s41393-018-0216-6. Epub 2018 Nov 9. PMID: 30413802.
5. Standaert C, Cardenas DD, Anderson P. Charcot spine as a late complication of traumatic spinal cord injury. Arch Phys Med Rehabil. 1997 Feb;78(2):221–225. doi: 10.1016/s0003-9993(97)90267-7. PMID: 9041906.

27 "It Hurts, and I'm Not Walking Right.": A Veteran with Back Pain and a Below Knee Prosthesis

Mary S. Keszler, David C. Morgenroth, Ari Greis, Rhonda M. Williams, Christopher J. Standaert

A 40-year-old Veteran of the US Armed Forces ("veteran") comes to your clinic due to progressive low back pain (LBP). Their history is notable for a traumatic injury to their right leg while deployed to a combat zone 15 years prior. This resulted in a right below knee amputation at the time of the injury. Your patient notes that prosthetic fitting has been a challenge, and they have not been seen for reevaluation of their prosthesis in over 5 years. They came in today because of low back pain that has come on over the last 6–12 months. Over the last 2 months, the pain has begun to radiate into their right anterior thigh. It particularly occurs with walking, and your patient notes it seems like their gait has gotten a bit more uneven. On examination, you note that they struggle a bit to walk with their prosthesis and that the right patellar reflex seems to be absent.

ow back pain (LBP) among people with limb loss (PWLL), is common; 52–76% of PWLL in the United States endorse LBP compared to a prevalence of approximately 30% in the general population. Rates of LBP are higher among those with transfemoral amputations (above knee) compared to transtibial amputations (below knee). PWLL can experience the same etiologies for LBP as those in the general population, but they have unique risk factors and presenting signs and symptoms to consider.

When evaluating LBP in PWLL, clinicians should consider intrinsic, prosthesis-related, and biopsychosocial factors. Intrinsic factors are related to limb loss etiology, associated trauma, and direct sequelae. In the setting of traumatic limb loss, it is important to ascertain the nature of the trauma (e.g. burn, blast, electrocution) and any associated injuries such as traumatic brain injury, spinal cord injury, or plexopathy. Furthermore, individuals with limb trauma may have had limb salvage attempted prior to their amputation. In such a scenario, the rehabilitation course can be complicated and prolonged with increased risk of deconditioning, joint contractures, and biopsychosocial sequelae (e.g. adjustment disorder due to new disability, post-traumatic stress disorder (PTSD), and anxiety, all of which are risk factors for LBP). Although uncommon, individuals with traumatic transfemoral amputations are also at risk of developing abdominal aortic aneurysms due to changes in distal blood flow, which could present as acute LBP.

For PWLL using a prosthesis, common gait and postural abnormalities, such as gait asymmetries, excessive lumbar spinal motion, and leg-length discrepancies can be associated with LBP. Inadequate socket fit and prosthetic alignment can exacerbate these issues. Optimizing the prosthesis (working with the patient's prosthetist) is therefore an important consideration.

Biopsychosocial factors are critical to consider when evaluating and treating LBP in PWLL. For instance, it is important to clarify how the amputation and LBP impact psychological health, mood, and social participation (e.g. relationships, employment status, recreational activities) and how these psychosocial factors may impact physical function. Veterans with traumatic amputation have a significantly higher rate of PTSD compared to those without traumatic limb loss, as well as elevated risk for depressive disorders. LBP in PWLL has also been associated with anxiety and kinesiophobia. Patients should be screened for health behaviors and sleep impairments which could exacerbate their pain. Cognitive impairment, poor health literacy, depression or low motivation, reduced self-advocacy, and systems-level factors (such as limited health care access and a suboptimal or absent working rapport with their prosthetist) can all impair prosthesis management, health, and function and potentially contribute to LBP.

Similar to anyone with LBP, PWLL should be screened for red flags like fever, incontinence, and unintentional weight loss that could be associated with serious underlying pathology. The history should include screening for biopsychosocial factors as described above. It is important to consider changes that may correspond temporally with symptoms (e.g. new life role or activity that may have occurred at the time of LBP onset). When evaluating prosthesis use, it is important to clarify the frequency and duration of use and any barriers, such as pain, poor fit or function, poor balance, falls, and use of gait aids.

When PWLL and LBP endorse new onset residual limb and/or phantom limb pain, a nerve root process or radiculopathy should be considered. The patient may describe pain radiating into the residual limb and sometimes into the phantom limb (depending on the spinal nerve root affected and the amputation level). LBP and radicular pain may impact sleep and quality of life, result in changes in gait, use of a new assistive device, and reduction or even cessation in prosthesis use. As a result, LBP can have a greater impact on functional independence in PWLL compared to individuals without limb loss.

The physical examination should include a standard LBP assessment, including lower limb manual muscle testing, sensation, reflexes, and lumbar and hip range of motion. Certain modifications are needed when assessing PWLL. Knee extension and flexion in a transtibial amputee need to be assessed differently than might be typical given the shortened residual limb, for example. During manual muscle testing, the hands should be placed in the same position on both limbs to ensure an accurate side-to-side comparison. It is also important to note that the amputated limb may be somewhat weaker than the intact limb for reasons other than radiculopathy (e.g. gait compensation). Commonly tested muscles, joint motions, and dermatomes may be absent in PWLL, given the amputation, presenting a more limited range of options for neurologic exam. Clinicians need to focus on proximal motions like hip abduction and internal rotation to assess lower lumbosa-cral nerve roots.

Direct examination of spinal motion is also different in PWLL than in those without limb loss. While it may be possible to assess lumbar flexion and extension in a standing position for a prosthesis user with good balance, this may not be feasible in other PWLL. Certain special tests can be helpful with minimal or no modifications. A modified slump test for lower lumbosacral radicular pain can be performed while the patient sits with the prosthesis off. The patient is asked to slump their shoulders and head forward while the examiner brings the leg into 90 degrees of hip flexion and full knee extension. Useful for lower lumbosacral roots only, a positive test reproduces the person's leg pain.

Given the limitations that may be present on history and physical exam in PWLL, a higher premium must be placed on diagnostic imaging (i.e. magnetic resonance imaging (MRI)) or electrodiagnostic testing (nerve conduction studies and electromyography). Since it may not be possible to perform a complete neurological examination in PWLL, such studies should be considered early in the evaluation process if the diagnosis is uncertain. As with all patients, care must be taken to clearly correlate any findings on imaging with the clinical presentation given the high prevalence of "abnormalities" in asymptomatic individuals, including disc degeneration, disc herniations, and spinal stenosis.

The residual limb should be inspected for wounds, calluses, and tender areas, as these could indicate poor socket fit or prosthesis alignment. Tenderness to palpation on the soft tissues of the distal residual limb that elicits electrical or shooting pain or radiating pain into the phantom limb could indicate a painful neuroma. Any of these findings could result in limb pain when ambulating, leading to changes in gait and potentially LBP.

For ambulatory individuals, it is vital to examine posture and gait. Leg-length discrepancy (LLD) can be assessed by placing one's hands on the bilateral iliac crests while the patient is standing with their feet shoulder-width apart and weight equally distributed (see Figure 27.1). A small LLD (<1 cm) is common and typically inconsequential. However, a larger LLD should be corrected by the prosthetist unless necessary for clearing the prosthetic foot when walking or consistent with patient preference. The gait

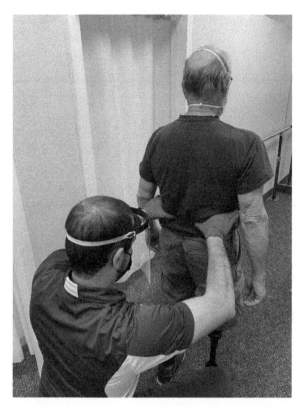

FIGURE 27.1. Examining for the leg length discrpency by comparing the position/ height of the iliac crests.

assessment should include evaluating the patient in the sagittal and coronal planes (i.e. with the examiner on the side of and in front of/behind the patient).

There are a few common gait deviations worth noting. An antalgic gait on the prosthetic side is characterized by reduced weight-bearing on the prosthetic limb while the other leg is swinging forward in the air. This typically indicates pain or discomfort on the amputated side. "Stepping into a hole" on the prosthetic side describes a gait deviation in which the hip on the prosthetic side drops lower than expected when stepping onto that leg. This typically indicates that the prosthesis is too short or the socket is too large or loose. PWLL can also commonly demonstrate difficulties clearing the prosthesis when swinging their limb forward, resulting in toe catching, tripping, and even falls. This can be due to the prosthesis being too long, the socket being too tight so the residual limb cannot fit into it properly, inadequate fit such that the prosthesis starts to slip off, or functionally weak hip abductors on the contralateral side leading to excessive hip drop on the prosthetic side.

In considering the case presented here, the leading diagnosis is an acute L3 or L4 radiculopathy in the setting of subacute to chronic LBP. Other potential etiologies could include degenerative spinal stenosis, degenerative spondylolisthesis, hip joint pathology, or meralgia paresthetica. The patient should be assessed for gait and prosthetic issues, as described above, to identify any problems that may be directly impacting gait and function of the lumbar spine. This is important in optimizing their outcome whatever else may arise during care.

Neurologic examination can be challenging. Dorsiflexion of the ankle is an important L4 function, but neither dorsiflexion nor the L4 dermatome (typically the distal medial calf) can be assessed. Relative hip weakness may be present, given the amputation, and the shortened tibia will limit assessment of knee extension strength (which can be affected by L3 or L4 radiculopathies). As such, it is difficult to identify an L4 radiculopathy (L5 and S1 nerve roots pose similar problems). The absent patellar reflex is enough to suggest a significant neurologic problem. Hip joint examination is relatively straight forward and should be performed. The residual limb should be examined for issues noted above, especially skin breakdown or a possible neuroma.

Given the limitations on exam, further objective diagnostic evaluation should be obtained, particularly plain radiographs of the lumbar spine with flexion/extension views, a lumbar spine MRI, and electrodiagnostic testing. As quadriceps weakness can be associated with substantial functional loss in an individual with a transtibial amputation, it is best to perform a thorough diagnostic evaluation promptly before embarking on a protracted care path. The patient here is 40 years old, making a lumbar disc herniation with an L3 or L4 radiculopathy the dominant diagnostic concern.

Assuming the diagnostic evaluation reveals findings consistent with a lumbar disc herniation with an L4 radiculopathy, there are a few distinct considerations that separate care for this patient from that for a patient without limb loss (see chapter 5 for a broader discussion of lumbar disc herniation). Initial decisions must consider the concern for progressive quadriceps or hip girdle weakness. Collaboration between surgical and non-surgical practitioners is important for this patient. If there is a sense that the patient is experiencing or at substantial risk for progressive weakness in their limb, surgery needs to be considered. If surgery is performed, it is important to recognize the potential functional implications of this in PWLL, such as transient change in functional independence and prosthesis use postoperatively due to activity restrictions and pain. There is also the risk of adverse outcomes following surgery, including pain, weakness, epidural fibrosis/arachnoiditis, or instability (see chapter 21). In the worst cases, these could lead to an inability to safely use a prosthesis. It is also important to bear in mind that fluid shifts associated with surgery can impact prosthesis fit postoperatively.

Assuming any weakness is minimal to mild and stable, it is reasonable to pursue nonoperative care. For this patient, physical therapy may be helpful for gait training, addressing hip or knee flexion contractures, hip girdle strength, and lumbar spine function. Standard over the counter analgesics can be used for pain. Consideration can be given to the use of oral corticosteroids or an epidural steroid injection for short-term pain relief.

If there are signs of mood or other psychiatric disorders such as PTSD, referral to a rehabilitation psychologist should be considered, given that there are empirically supported treatments available. It is important to treat these disorders to remission. This patient may also benefit from participation in amputee support groups, peer mentorship through the Amputee Coalition (a national, nonprofit organization for PWLL), or self-management courses, such as Promoting Amputee Life Skills through the Amputee Coalition. An important aspect of lifelong care for PWLL is ensuring regular care with their prosthetist (if they are a prosthesis user) and physiatrist. The physiatrist and prosthetist will ideally work together to address any prosthesis fit or function problems, which may be of benefit in the prevention and treatment of LBP.

1. PWLL are more likely to experience LBP during their lifetime than the general population.
2. LBP in PWLL is associated with PTSD, depression, and anxiety.
3. Inadequate rehabilitation, hip girdle and core weakness, joint contractures, poor prosthesis fit, and gait deviations could be contributing factors to developing LBP.
4. The physical exam associated with LBP typically needs to be modified in PWLL.
5. PWLL should maintain follow-up with their prosthetist and physiatrist.

Further reading

1. Czerniecki JM, Ehde DM. Chronic pain after lower extremity amputation. Crit Rev Phys Rehab Med. 2003;15(4):309–332.
2. Gailey R, Allen K, Castles J, Kucharik J, Roeder M. Review of secondary physical conditions associated with lower-limb amputation and long-term prosthesis use. J Rehabil Res Dev. 2008;45(1):15–29.
3. Highsmith MJ, Goff LM, Lewandowski A, Farrokhi S, Hendershot BD, Hill OT, et al. Low back pain in persons with lower extremity amputation: a systematic review of the literature. Spine J. 2019;19(3):552–563.
4. Mazzone B, Farrokhi S, Hendershot BD, McCabe CT, Watrous JR. Prevalence of low back pain and relationship to mental health symptoms and quality of life after a deployment-related lower limb amputation. Spine (Phila Pa 1976). 2020;45(19):1368–1375.
5. Morgenroth DC, Orendurff MS, Shakir A, Segal A, Shofer J, Czerniecki JM. The relationship between lumbar spine kinematics during gait and low-back pain in transfemoral amputees. Am J Phys Med Rehabil. 2010;89(8):635–643.

28 "I'm Only in My Second Trimester, but Now My Back Hurts.": Back Pain in Pregnancy

Jason S. Bitterman

A 28-year-old female comes into your clinic with concerns about back pain. She is currently 26 weeks pregnant. This is her first pregnancy, and she has been doing well until recently. She has been walking every day for exercise, watching her diet, and has appropriate weight gain thus far. Over the last couple of weeks, she has been having increasing lower back pain. It is painful when she walks but also if she sits for an extended time. There is some radiation into her left buttock and proximal posterior thigh. The pain disrupts her sleep at times. She has been trying heat and ice topically and her partner has been doing some gentle massage. Despite this, the pain has been worsening. She is clearly concerned.

What do you do now?

M ore than 50% of pregnant women experience low back pain (LBP). While back pain is often considered a normal phenomenon in pregnancy, health care providers should not neglect these symptoms, as they can significantly impact women's lives. Over half of pregnant women with low back and pelvic pain report difficulty with activities of daily living, and it is one of the main causes for sick leave during pregnancy.

The definition of "pregnancy-related back pain" is ambiguous in the medical literature and is sometimes used as a catch-all for any type of back or pelvic pain during pregnancy. "Pregnancy-related back pain" is an umbrella term for two different entities: pregnancy-related low back pain (PLBP) and pelvic girdle pain (PGP). These disorders have different presentations, although they often occur together. Clinicians should be mindful of why PLBP and PGP occur, the differential diagnosis, the treatment options, and the prognosis.

The cause of PLBP and PGP is not fully understood. It is likely due to a series of biomechanical changes. Joint laxity is frequently considered the primary cause of back pain in pregnancy. Studies have found patients with pregnancy-related back pain demonstrate increased pelvic motion compared to asymptomatic pregnant women. Poor stability likely causes increased stress on pelvic and lumbar spine structures, such as joints, ligaments, and the surrounding musculature. This laxity is often attributed to the hormone relaxin. Relaxin induces collagen remodeling, which was theorized to increase pelvic laxity and widening of the pubic symphysis. However, recent studies have not found a relationship between relaxin levels and increased pelvic mobility or peripheral joint mobility.

The enlarging gravid uterus also causes several biomechanical changes that can potentially result in back pain. As a pregnancy progresses, the patient's center of gravity shifts anteriorly, causing an anterior pelvic tilt. This predisposes the patient to a hyperlordotic posture, which increases load on the axial skeleton. In combination with increased pelvic laxity, anterior pelvic tilt also increases stress on structures of the pelvis, especially the sacroiliac (SI) joints. Finally, the enlarged gravid uterus can stretch and weaken the abdominal muscles. This can reduce core abdominal strength, leading to less muscular support of the axial spine. All the above biomechanical changes increase strain on the lumbar spine and pelvis, leading to PLBP and PGP.

PLBP and PGP rarely occur before 18 weeks of gestation, and both peak between 24 and 36 weeks. This is likely because many of the biomechanical changes are caused by the enlarged gravid uterus from the mid-second trimester through the third trimester.

PLBP and PGP tend to have different presentations. PLBP presents with pain in the low back region above the sacrum. The pain may radiate to the posterior buttocks and thighs. This pain is typically worse with lumbar flexion activities. These patients tend to have restricted lumbar range of motion.

PGP is more common than PLBP. These patients have pain in the posterior pelvis (between the posterior iliac crest and gluteal folds). The pain may radiate to the posterior thighs. There may also be concomitant anterior pelvic pain at the pubic symphysis with radiation to the anterior thighs. The pain can be exacerbated by various activities, including walking, standing, sitting, twisting, unequal weight-bearing on one leg, and turning in bed. There is typically no restricted lumbar range of motion. PGP patients are usually more debilitated and have more difficulty performing activities of daily living compared to PLBP patients.

When examining a pregnant woman with back pain, clinicians should do a thorough lumbar spine exam, hip exam, and lower limb neurologic exam. Patients with PLBP and PGP should have no focal neurologic deficits.

While PLBP and PGP are the most common causes of back pain in pregnancy, clinicians must be mindful of other causes of LBP (Table 28.1). All patients should be screened for red flag signs and symptoms that may be indicative of cauda equina syndrome, malignancy, or infection. PLBP and PGP do not cause any red flag symptoms, and positive findings warrant urgent investigation. Lumbar disc herniations can occur in pregnancy. However, pregnancy alone does not increase the risk of a disc herniation. Only 2% of pregnant patients with a disc herniation develop cauda equina syndrome or significant neurologic deficit. Rarely, pregnancy can cause osteoporosis, usually in the third trimester or just after delivery, which in turn can cause a vertebral compression fracture. This should be considered in women in their third trimester with sudden, severe back pain in the thoracic or lumbar region.

PLBP and PGP are clinical diagnoses. No additional testing is necessary if other diagnoses are unlikely. Imaging should be obtained if the history

TABLE 28.1 **Differential Diagnosis for Low Back Pain in Pregnancy**

Lumbar Spine Pathology

Pregnancy-related low back pain (PLBP)

Lumbar disc herniation

Lumbar radiculopathy

Lumbar spondylosis

Cauda equina syndrome

Vertebral compression fracture

Spondylolysis/spondylolisthesis

Osteomyelitis/discitis

Pelvic Pathology

Pelvic girdle pain (PGP)

Sacroiliac joint laxity

Osteitis pubis

Rupture of symphysis pubis

Obstetric Pathology

Preterm labor

Placental abruption

Round ligament pain

Chorioamnionitis

Other

Neoplasm (e.g. spinal tumor, pelvic tumor)

Urinary tract infection

Pyelonephritis

Ankylosing spondylitis

and exam are suggestive of cauda equina syndrome or malignancy or if the patient has persistent severe pain despite conservative management. The imaging modality of choice for pregnant women with LBP, when necessary, is a lumbar or pelvic MRI. This can be used to identify disc herniations with potential nerve root compression and central canal stenosis, spinal tumors, symptomatic vertebral hemangiomas, SI joint edema, vertebral fractures, and sacral stress fractures. In terms of safety, there is debate whether MRIs can cause fetal teratogenicity and acoustic damage, particularly with 3-Tesla MRIs (MRI magnets typically range from 0.5 to 3 Tesla in strength). Because of this, some recommend delaying MRIs until after the first trimester. MRIs should not be performed with contrast, as gadolinium can be dangerous for the developing fetus, and most causes of LBP do not require contrast for diagnosis.

Plain radiographs (X-ray) and computed tomography (CT) imaging should be avoided as ionizing radiation can cause spontaneous abortions, intrauterine growth restriction, and fetal malformations. These may be indicated after serious trauma. Ultrasound, while safe, does not provide sufficient information for lumbar spine and SI joint pathologies to be of use.

Women with PLBP and PGP should be treated conservatively. Patient education and counseling is critical, as the pain can significantly impact patients' lives while they may also have other pregnancy-related symptoms and stressors. PBLP and PGP are usually self-limiting conditions. However, a small number of patients have persistent symptoms for weeks, months, and potentially years after delivery. PGP tends to have a worse prognosis compared to PBLP. Risk factors for long-term symptoms include prepregnancy LBP, prolonged labor duration, severity of pain during pregnancy, low mobility, and inability to return to prepregnancy weight following delivery.

Physical therapy should be prescribed in women with PLBP and potentially those with PGP. There is some evidence that exercise in pregnant patients with LBP can reduce pain, disability, and time taken for sick leave. The evidence for exercise programs is not as strong for pregnant women with pelvic pain alone. Physical therapy should aim to teach patients comfortable positioning (during sleep, sitting, etc.) and exercises that compensate for the biomechanical changes that occur in pregnancy.

There is limited evidence for other conservative treatments, although they may be considered in patients with refractory pain. Pelvic belts have been used for patients with both PLBP and PGP. These are thought to reduce SI joint and pubic symphysis instability and better disperse force to the back and pelvic girdle, which may provide relief. Patients should be instructed to wear pelvic belts around the greater trochanters and to use them for short periods at a time. Aquatic exercise, yoga, and massage are also potential treatment options, although the evidence for these is limited. For nighttime pain, patients should be encouraged to try different pillows to support both their back and abdomen.

Acetaminophen has traditionally been the first-line analgesic in pregnancy. However, recent evidence suggests it may alter fetal development, and it should be used with caution. Nonsteroidal anti-inflammatory drugs should be avoided due to the risk of premature closure of the ductus arteriosus. Opioids are not recommended.

Nonsurgical interventions are rarely performed for pregnancy-related LBP. Epidural steroid injections are unlikely to treat PLBP and PGP. They may only be of utility in a patient with a severe acute lumbar radiculopathy that has not responded to conservative treatments. Note that this procedure generally requires fluoroscopic or CT guidance, which can expose the fetus to ionizing radiation.

Surgery is reserved for pregnant patients with progressive neurologic deficits or cauda equina syndrome. These most commonly are due to a disc herniation or mass. Surgery carries serious potential risks to both the mother and fetus due to patient positioning and anesthetics. The surgery may also induce a preterm labor. If possible, surgery should be delayed until after delivery. Surgical planning requires close coordination between an obstetrician, surgeon, anesthesiologist, and neonatologist.

Clinicians should educate patients, particularly those with PGP, of the prognosis and closely follow them not just during pregnancy but postpartum as well. Counseling, exercise, oral medications, and other therapies for back and pelvic pain should continue to be used to treat these patients.

For our 28-year-old pregnant patient with LBP, she had restricted lumbar flexion on exam with pain and was diagnosed with PLBP. We prescribed a course of physical therapy. She did her lumbopelvic core stability exercises daily. She also trialed a pelvic belt, which helped her tolerate walking on days when her pain was significant. After 4 weeks, her pain was better controlled and she was more comfortable for the remainder of her pregnancy.

1. LBP and pelvic pain are very common during pregnancy and tend to be self-limiting, but they should not be treated with benign neglect. All patients should have a thorough evaluation.
2. Clinicians should distinguish between PLBP and PGP as their presentations and prognoses are different, which can help guide patient education and setting expectations. Typically, PGP is more severe and more likely to persist postpartum.
3. Clinicians should consider other causes of LBP, especially in patients with intractable pain or neurologic abnormalities.
4. PLBP and PGP are clinical diagnoses. Imaging should only be ordered if other diagnoses, such as cauda equina syndrome or malignancy, are acute clinical concerns.
5. PBLP and PGP should be treated conservatively with patient education, counseling, and physical therapy. Pelvic belts and other complementary treatments may be considered.

Further reading

1. Liddle SD, Pennick V. Interventions for preventing and treating low-back and pelvic pain during pregnancy. Cochrane Database Syst Rev. 2015;2015(9):1–28.
2. Sehmbi H, D'Souza R, Bhatia A. Low back pain in pregnancy: investigations, management, and role of neuraxial analgesia and anaesthesia: a systematic review. Gynecol Obstet Invest. 2017;82(5):417–436.
3. Shiri R, Coggon D, Falah-Hassani K. Exercise for the prevention of low back and pelvic girdle pain in pregnancy: a meta-analysis of randomized controlled trials. Eur J Pain. 2018;22(1):19–27.
4. Vermani E, Mittal R, Weeks A. Pelvic girdle pain and low back pain in pregnancy: a review. Pain Pract. 2010;10(1):60–71.
5. Wuytack F, Begley C, Daly D. Risk factors for pregnancy-related pelvic girdle pain: a scoping review. BMC Pregnancy Childbirth. 2020;20(1):739.

29 "I Didn't Think This Third Pregnancy Was Going to Be So Hard on Me.": A 33-Year-Old with Postpartum Pelvic Pain

Marissa L. Marcotte, Rupali Kumar

A 33-year-old female (gravida 3 para 3) who is 4 months postpartum presents with low back pain (LBP) since her third trimester of pregnancy. She is a single mother whose first child, age 5, was born via vaginal delivery, and second child, age 2, was born via cesarean section (C-section). She had gestational diabetes with her latest pregnancy and tried to undergo a vaginal birth after cesarean (VBAC). C-section was pursued after failure to progress. She began walking around her block 2 weeks after delivery, as recommended by her obstetrician, but has been busy and fatigued with her newborn and two other children. Her sleep is poor, and she struggles to find the energy she had hoped for at this point. Over the last month, her activity has been hampered further by pain across her low back that radiates a bit into her left buttock. It hurts to lift things, including her children, or if she is on her feet for 30 minutes. She is nursing her newborn and is concerned about taking medications.

What do you do now?

ow back pain (LBP) during pregnancy and in the postpartum period is extremely common. Compared to LBP in the general population, in which lumbar sources of pain are the most common, pregnant and postpartum patients tend to experience pain in the pelvic girdle. The pelvic girdle is a bony structure of 3 fused bones (ilium, ischium, and pubis) that articulate at the pubic symphysis anteriorly and the sacroiliac (SI) joints posteriorly. Posterior pelvic girdle pain from the SI joint can radiate to the buttock and posterior thigh but does not go past the knee.

The differential diagnosis for LBP in pregnancy and postpartum includes musculotendinous or ligamentous sources, pelvic stress fractures, femoral stress fractures, and transient osteoporosis of pregnancy (particularly with tailbone pain), while radiating pain down the leg can be due to lumbosacral radiculopathy (potentially related to disc pathology), plexopathy, sciatic neuropathy, or meralgia paresthetica. In this population, a history of pain in the low back that radiates to the buttock and posterior thigh and increases with walking, transitional movements, and prolonged standing, is suggestive of pelvic girdle pain from an SI joint origin, as opposed to what is more commonly thought of as "sciatica" or radicular pain arising in the lumbar spine.

Posterior pelvic pain in pregnancy and postpartum is unique from LBP in the general population due to the contribution of hormonal and biomechanical changes that result from pregnancy and delivery. Estrogen, progesterone, and relaxin promote ligamentous laxity to help accommodate the growing fetus and prepare for delivery, and the resulting instability can lead to pain. The biomechanical effects of this laxity are compounded by 20–30-pound weight gain, enlargement in breasts and uterus, and anterior displacement of the center of mass. This shifted center of mass magnifies forces on the joints and leads to postural changes, functional impairment, and pain. Hormonal and biomechanical changes continue into the postpartum period, as well, particularly if one is breastfeeding. Posterior pelvic girdle pain is often worse and appears earlier with each successive pregnancy. This hypermobility-induced pain is compounded by the repetitive motion involved in taking care of infants and small children, with repeated bending, lifting, and prolonged carrying.

In this patient's case, the presence of gestational diabetes likely contributed to a higher birthweight baby, and the increased weight could have intensified the biomechanical issues noted above. In addition, abdominal weakness is often noted in the pregnant and postpartum state, with stretching of abdominal muscles out of a position of mechanical advantage, as well as rectus diastasis (separation in the rectus abdominis muscles) contributing to core weakness. This is further exacerbated in C-section delivery with incision through the abdominal muscles causing functional weakness and pain. Patients undergoing C-sections are generally under-rehabilitated for the extent of the associated trauma.

Treating patients with pain from SI joint or pelvic origin starts with education. After a thorough exam to rule out any neurological changes, you can reassure the patient that although they are experiencing radiating pain, they do not have any nerve damage such as with lumbar radiculopathy or sciatic neuropathy. Their symptoms can be managed conservatively with physical therapy, which can provide improved function in addition to pain relief. Goals with physical therapy include improving simple biomechanics/ergonomics (work, activities of daily living (ADLs), breastfeeding, and childcare). Rehabilitation can focus on strengthening exercises to promote trunk and pelvic stabilization, muscle energy techniques, soft tissue mobilization, and stretching (buttocks, hamstrings, quadratus lumborum, iliopsoas). Encourage patients to wear proper supportive footwear, as hormonal changes on the ligaments in the feet can lead to flattened arches. Many women will also experience immediate improvement from a sacroiliac joint stability belt.

Generally speaking, many over the counter analgesics are safe and effective at managing this kind of pain while therapy is ongoing. However, distinct concerns arise in those who are pregnant or nursing. With patients who are breastfeeding or pumping, consider possible medication exposure to the baby from breastmilk. Regarding analgesics, first-line agents include acetaminophen and nonsteroidal anti-inflammatory drugs (NSAIDs) in the postpartum mother. While they should be avoided in pregnancy, NSAIDs have limited uptake into breastmilk and can safely be used in the postpartum period. Safe options include ibuprofen, indomethacin, and naproxen. Lidocaine patches can be used for localized pain, although they may be less effective over areas with greater amounts of subcutaneous tissue.

It is important to note that while LBP is *common* during pregnancy and in the postpartum period, one should be cautious to not write off the pain as being "expected" or even "normal," and thus fail to address it. Unfortunately, some practitioners may cite limited workup or treatment options during the perinatal period, or simply decide to "watch and wait" until after delivery or after the patient is no longer breastfeeding. Failing to treat back pain in these individuals has significant repercussions on sleep, mood, job productivity, and social interaction, and can predispose patients to persistent, chronic pain.

There is a strong correlation between worsened pain and mood disorders such as depression and anxiety. This chapter will focus on the unique differences for diagnosing and treating postpartum women experiencing depressed mood, but much of the management will use the same multidisciplinary approach as depression in the general population (LBP and depression are discussed further in chapter 17).

Postpartum depression (PPD) has the same diagnostic criteria as major depression, requiring at least five of nine symptoms for at least 2 weeks: depressed mood, loss of interest, lack of sleep, change in weight/appetite disturbance, fatigue, agitation/motor slowing, feelings of worthlessness/guilt, decreased concentration, and suicidal thoughts. It is one of the most common complications of childbirth. Onset of PPD can happen between 4 weeks and 12 months after childbirth. The strongest risk factor is history of mood or anxiety disorder at any point in life, especially if symptomatic in pregnancy. There is also an increased risk with history of gestational diabetes, higher maternal age, poor social support, shorter gestational age, stressful life events, poor quality of marital relationship, low socioeconomic status, low self-esteem, and unplanned or unwanted pregnancy. This patient has at least three of these risk factors, including gestational diabetes, higher maternal age, and poor social support. Importantly, PPD can have consequences on all members of the family, not just the mother.

PPD is separate from "postpartum blues" which is a mild and transient syndrome (less than 2 weeks) of low mood, tearfulness, and mild irritability that does not impair function. More than 50% of women have postpartum blues shortly after childbirth. If symptoms persist, it is possible for postpartum blues to transition to PPD. Screening tools to identify PPD include the Edinburg Postnatal Depression Scale (EPDS), Patient Health Questionnaire-9 (PHQ-9), and the Beck Depression Inventory. A benefit to the EPDS is that it measures mood-related symptoms (ability to laugh, guilt, feeling overwhelmed), rather than somatic symptoms (lack of sleep, fatigue, change in appetite) that may be associated with pregnancy and delivery.

Treatment for PPD should have a multidisciplinary and stepwise approach depending upon the severity of symptoms. Starting with psychological interventions, strategies should be implemented to increase self-care, improve social support, and reduce the occurrence and impact of negative life events or stressors. Psychotherapy options include cognitive behavioral therapy (CBT), interpersonal psychotherapy (IPT), listening visits, and supportive counseling. If mood is being impacted by lack of sleep, differentiate between the patient not being able to sleep when the baby is sleeping vs. insomnia due to infant care. If the patient is limited by the child's sleep patterns, targeting infant sleep interventions can lead to improvement in maternal sleep. This can be achieved with the help of medical providers trained in infant sleep or seeking resources online. Helpful strategies include developing bedtime routines and putting the infant to sleep in a safe environment while awake, without parental intervention. If the child sleeps well and the mother is still having issues with sleep, this may be an indicator of mood disorder. Overall, sleep is important to address, as poor sleep, especially in the setting of mood disorder, can lead to worsened pain.

In cases of severe PPD not responsive to conservative psychological interventions, medication management and/or electroconvulsive therapy can be considered. Most antidepressants are not contraindicated during breastfeeding or pumping due to minimal uptake into breastmilk. Serotonin reuptake inhibitors (SSRIs) are the first-line antidepressant medications for PPD treatment due to low toxicity risk in setting of potential overdose and less severe side effects. Among the SSRIs, sertraline has been found to have the least passage into breastmilk, and is thus often preferred for mothers. If SSRIs are ineffective, mirtazapine, or serotonin norepinephrine reuptake inhibitors (SNRIs), such as duloxetine and venlafaxine, also appear to have minimal passage into breastmilk. An alternative antidepressant can be used, especially in the setting of controlled mood when used prior to pregnancy.

It is not clear whether any specific antidepressant is more effective than another for treatment of PPD. Other classes of antidepressants have less information on lactation exposure. Bupropion should be avoided if possible due to some reports of infant seizure. Tricyclic antidepressants (TCAs) have greater passage into breastmilk than SSRIs and have a high risk for potential overdose. If TCAs must be used, nortriptyline is believed to be safest. Doxepin (a TCA) is contraindicated due to adverse events reported in infants. Additional precautions before starting medications should be used in the setting where the child was delivered prematurely or is medically ill. These conversations can be had with the child's pediatrician. If needed, mothers can consider switching to formula feeding their baby.

Electroconvulsive therapy (ECT) is an option in treating severe PPD, especially if the patient is suicidal or if there are concomitant psychotic symptoms. However, it requires a general anesthetic and can have side effects, such as memory impairment.

Overall, this patient likely has posterior pelvic pain originating from the SI joint. This is a common source of pain due to ligamentous laxity and subsequent joint instability experienced in pregnancy and the postpartum period. Improvement in pain and function can be achieved with conservative management including physical therapy and over the counter analgesics, such as acetaminophen and ibuprofen. If there are any signs of postpartum depression, this should be managed as well, because depression can cause worsened pain symptoms. Furthermore, postpartum depression can negatively impact all members of the family, not just the mother.

KEY POINTS

1. Hormonal changes leading to ligamentous laxity and joint instability with subsequent biomechanical changes are the most common underlying etiology of LBP in pregnant and postpartum women.
2. Radiating LBP to the buttock and thigh is more typically related to the posterior pelvic girdle and SI joint in this population and less commonly radicular in origin.

3. LBP in this population is worsened due to the repetitive motions associated with childcare.
4. Postpartum depression treatment is similar to the general population and includes a multidisciplinary approach with psychotherapy and medications if needed.
5. Postpartum depression is important to treat as it can worsen pain symptoms.

Further reading

1. Reese ME, Casey E. "Hormonal Influence on the Neuromusculoskeletal System in Pregnancy." In *Musculoskeletal Health in Pregnancy and Postpartum*, edited by C Fitzgerald, N Segal. Cham: Springer, 2015:19–39.
2. Segal NA, Chu SR. "Musculoskeletal Anatomic, Gait, and Balance Changes in Pregnancy and Risk for Falls." In *Musculoskeletal Health in Pregnancy and Postpartum*, edited by C Fitzgerald, N Segal. Cham: Springer, 2015:1–18.
3. Stewart DE, Vigod SN. Postpartum depression: pathophysiology, treatment, and emerging therapeutics. Annu Rev Med. 2019 Jan 27;70:183–196. doi: 10.1146/annurev-med-041217-011106. PMID: 30691372.
4. Centers for Disease Control and Prevention. Breastfeeding: prescription medication use. Accessed 12/1/2022. cdc.gov/breastfeeding/breastfeeding-special-circumstances/vaccinations-medications-drugs/prescription-medication-use.html.

30 "It Really Hurts When I Get Up.": A 24-Year-Old Male with Progressive Sacral Pain and Stiffness

Niveditha Mohan

A 24-year-old male comes to see you for increasing back pain. Over the past 12 months, he has noted gradually worsening low back pain (LBP) and stiffness. He initially attributed it to running for exercise, which he uses to manage long-standing anxiety. He cut back and then stopped running about 6 months ago, but the pain has persisted and progressed. He now has discomfort that sometimes wakes him up at night, and he is more anxious. He feels very stiff, particularly in the morning for 2–3 hours and after he has been sitting for even a short amount of time, he needs to get up, walk, and stretch frequently to feel relief. He saw a chiropractor but benefits last only for a few hours after each treatment. He has no leg pain or numbness. He is very healthy otherwise with no prior history of back problems. He has tried over the counter nonsteroidal anti-inflammatory drugs (NSAID) with minimal and temporary benefit. Heat and ice do not help. He is getting quite desperate to figure this out.

What do you do now?

A mong patients who present in primary care settings for LBP, approximately 0.5% will have an inflammatory etiology for the pain, such as axial spondyloarthritis (axSpA). Characteristics that suggest an inflammatory etiology include morning stiffness lasting more than an hour, improvement with exercise (gelling phenomenon), and pain at night. AxSpA is a potentially disabling inflammatory arthritis of the spine, usually presenting as chronic LBP, typically before the age of 45. It can be associated with one or more articular (synovitis), periarticular (enthesitis, dactylitis), or extraarticular features (uveitis, psoriasis, inflammatory bowel disease). There are two subtypes of axSpA: ankylosing spondylitis (AS, also termed radiographic axSpA) and nonradiographic axSpA (nr-axSpA). The former typically presents with features of sacroiliitis and/or lumbar spine involvement on X-rays, and the latter does not have definite radiographic changes but does have clinical symptoms of inflammatory LBP and other features associated with axSpA.

AS is more common among men, but nr-axSpA is equally distributed among men and women. Because the majority (70%) of patients in early disease will not have definite radiographic changes at the time of diagnosis, the Assessment of SpondyloArthritis International Society (ASAS) classification criteria were developed for patients with back pain greater than 3 months and age of onset <45 years. Patients are divided into those who have HLA-B27 positivity plus >2 other SpA features or sacroiliitis on imaging plus >1 SpA feature (see Table 30.1). HLA-B27 positivity is seen in over 90% of White AS patients and 50–80% of non-White AS patients. However, the HLA-B27 allele is seen in 6–9% of healthy whites and 3% of healthy North American Black patients. Since the overall prevalence of AS in the general US population is 0.5%, only 2% (1 in 50) of HLA-B27 positive individuals develop AS during their lifetime. Hence most patients with AS can be diagnosed based on history, physical exam, and the findings of sacroiliitis on X-rays, obviating the need for HLA testing. HLA-B27 is hypothesized to play a role in the pathogenesis of AS through various mechanisms but has not proven useful as a therapeutic target.

TABLE 30.1 Diagnostic Features and Imaging Findings in Spondyloarthritis

Spondyloarthritis (SpA) Features	Sacroiliitis Imaging
· Inflammatory back pain · Arthritis · Enthesitis (heel) · Uveitis · Dactylitis · Psoriasis · Crohn's/colitis · Good response to NSAIDs · Family history of SpA · HLA-B27 · Elevated CRP	· Active (acute) inflammation on MRI highly suggestive of sacroiliitis associated with SpA · Definite radiographic sacroiliitis according to modified NY criteria

Major musculoskeletal features include the following:

a) Inflammatory back pain of >3 months duration with insidious onset, improvement with exercise but not with rest, pain at night, and good response to anti-inflammatory doses of analgesics.

b) Peripheral arthritis—about 35–40% of patients with axSpA have an associated peripheral arthritis predominantly in the knees and ankles, asymmetrical, oligoarticular (1–3 joints).

c) Enthesitis—this refers to inflammation around the enthesis, which is the insertion of ligaments, tendons, joint capsule, or fascia to bone and is relatively specific to SpA. The most commonly affected areas include the Achilles tendon and plantar fascia, but any other area of tendon/ligament insertion can also develop pain and tenderness.

d) Dactylitis (sausage digits)—this is a characteristic feature of SpA; and unlike synovitis where the swelling is confined to the joints, with dactylitis, the entire digit is swollen due to swelling in the flexor tendon sheath and marked adjacent soft tissue involvement.

Major non-musculoskeletal features include the following:

a) Inflammatory eye disease—conjunctivitis and anterior uveitis are the most common. The former is typically non-purulent and transient. Patients with uveitis present with redness, pain, and photophobia. Episodes of uveitis do not always parallel the course of the musculoskeletal manifestations.

b) Inflammatory bowel disease—prevalence of inflammatory bowel disease among patients with AS is 6.8%.

c) Psoriasis—is seen in up to 10% of patients with AS.

d) Aortic insufficiency (3–10%), ascending aortitis, and other cardiac manifestations such as conduction abnormalities, diastolic dysfunction, pericarditis, and ischemic heart disease have been described.

e) Pulmonary manifestations include upper lobe fibrosis and restrictive changes.

A complete physical exam is necessary to elucidate both articular and extraarticular manifestations of the disease. However, there are specific physical examination tests that can be useful to assess sacroiliac joint tenderness or progression of spinal disease in axSpA patients. They include:

- Occiput to wall test assesses loss of cervical range of motion. In normal individuals, standing with heels and scapulae touching the wall, the occiput should also touch the wall. Any distance from the occiput to the wall represents a forward stoop of the neck secondary to cervical spine involvement.

- Chest expansion detects chest mobility. Normal chest expansion is about 5 cm and anything less than 2.5 cm is considered abnormal.

- Schober test (modified) detects limitation of forward flexion of the lumbar spine. Place a mark at the level of the posterior superior iliac spine (dimples of Venus) and another 10 cm above the midline. With maximal forward spinal flexion with locked knees, the measured distance should increase from 10 cm to at least 15 cm.

- Patrick's test assesses sacroiliac joint tenderness. With the patient's heel placed on the opposite knee, downward pressure on the flexed knee with the hip now in flexion, abduction, and external rotation (FABER) should elicit contralateral sacroiliac joint tenderness.

Laboratory studies are frequently obtained in patients suspected of having axSpA, particularly HLA-B27. Given the high prevalence of positivity in the general population, a positive HLA-B27 by itself is not diagnostic of

AS. Conversely, a negative HLA-B27 does not exclude the diagnosis either. It should be used judiciously in those who have inflammatory symptoms without radiographic changes to decide whether they make criteria for nr-axSpA and are candidates for treatment. Erythrocyte sedimentation rate (ESR) and levels of C-reactive protein (CRP) are increased in 35–50% of patients with AS.

Imaging is the cornerstone in the diagnosis of axSpA. Plain radiographs of the lumbar spine and sacroiliac (SI) joints should be obtained. In early disease, radiographs can be normal. However, findings consistent with sacroiliitis, syndesmophytes, and bamboo spine are suggestive of long-standing AS. Peripheral radiographs can also show erosive changes in the joints and signs of enthesitis (fluffy calcification at sites of tendon insertions with erosions). In those patients with inflammatory features but negative radiographs, MRI of the lumbar spine and SI joints may show periarticular bone marrow edema which, when interpreted with clinical findings, can help make the diagnosis of axSpA.

Goals and general principles of management include the relief of symptoms, maintenance of function, prevention of complications of spinal disease, minimization of extraarticular manifestations and comorbidities, and maintenance of effective psychosocial functioning. Since this is a chronic disease that affects younger individuals, it is important to educate patients about the prognosis and risks and benefits of recommended interventions. Physical therapy and exercise are key to maintaining function and long-term productivity. Smoking cessation should be encouraged and supported to minimize the effect on pulmonary function. In addition to control of disease activity, symptoms that require recognition and appropriate treatment include anxiety, depression, fatigue, sleep disturbance, and helplessness, which also contribute to functional limitations in some patients with axSpA.

A range of pharmacological treatment options exist for patients with axSpA. The choice of therapy is based on the selection of agents that would be effective for the clinical manifestations in that individual patient. Nonsteroidal anti-inflammatory drugs (NSAIDs) are the standard initial therapy in most patients with symptomatic axSpA. Regardless of the NSAID used, the maximum dose is often required. The potential gastrointestinal, renal, cardiovascular, and other risks of NSAIDs need to be considered when using these agents. About 70–80% of AS patients report substantial relief of their symptoms with NSAIDs. Duration of NSAID use is determined by length of symptoms and extent of response. If the patient requires continuous use or has inadequate response to initial therapy with two different NSAIDs used consecutively for at least 2–4 weeks each, other treatment interventions are recommended.

Unfortunately, none of the traditional disease modifying anti-rheumatic drugs (DMARDs) that work for other inflammatory arthritides, such as methotrexate and leflunomide, work to suppress inflammation involving the spine. Tumor necrosis factor (TNF) inhibitors have been ground-breaking in this regard and have been shown to prevent disease progression with symptom control in many patients. Contraindications to use of these agents include active infection, latent/untreated tuberculosis, demyelinating disease (e.g. multiple sclerosis, optic neuritis), heart failure, and certain malignancies. Interleukin 17 (IL-17) inhibitors can have a role in treatment, and secukinumab/Ixekizumab (anti-IL-17A monoclonal antibody) is an alternative to TNF inhibitors for patients with axSpA. Tofacitibib and upadacitinib are janus kinase (JAK) inhibitors that have been approved for the treatment of AS. These agents carry an increased risk of cardiovascular disease, blood clots, and cancer and should be used only if the patient fails TNF or IL-17 inhibitors with careful monitoring.

Treatment for the patient presented here should be based on his response to NSAIDs at full anti-inflammatory dosing and the results of blood tests and imaging studies, which should include radiographs of SI joint and lumbar spine. He should be started on an initial trial of full dose NSAIDs for 2–4 weeks. If he has an excellent response, NSAIDs can be used as needed. If he has an inadequate response or has radiographic changes, he should be started on a TNF inhibitor after discussion of risks and benefits and prescreening for hepatitis, tuberculosis, and human immunodeficiency virus. Once his symptoms are under good control (typically 6 weeks after starting a TNF inhibitor), he should start physical therapy for back strengthening and conditioning. Concomitantly with above pharmacological interventions, he should be advised against smoking and associated psychosocial issues such as depression and anxiety should be addressed to optimize his ability to maintain full function.

1. Inflammatory back pain should be distinguished from mechanical back pain; if pain has been present for more than 3 months in a younger individual, AS should be considered in the differential diagnosis.
2. Both articular and extraarticular manifestations should be assessed in the history and physical examination.
3. Early axSpA may not have radiographic findings, and MRI may be necessary to find objective evidence of inflammation in the sacroiliac and spine joints.
4. Treatment should be individualized based on the presenting manifestations in that specific patient.
5. Non-pharmacological interventions are critical to maintain physical and psychosocial functioning in these patients.

Further reading

1. Rudwaleit M, van der Heijde D, Landewé R, et al. The Assessment of Spondyloarthritis International Society classification criteria for peripheral spondyloarthritis and for spondyloarthritis in general. Ann Rheum Dis. 2011;70:25.
2. El Maghraoui A. Extra-articular manifestations of ankylosing spondylitis: prevalence, characteristics, and therapeutic implications. Eur J Intern Med. 2011;22:554.
3. van der Heijde D, Ramiro S, Landewé R, et al. 2016 update of the ASAS-EULAR management recommendations for axial spondyloarthritis. Ann Rheum Dis. 2017;76:978.

31 "My Hip Hurts.": Is It Her Back?

Isaiah Levy, Christopher J. Standaert

You are seeing a 54-year-old patient. When you ask how you can help her today, she states, "My hip hurts." The pain is on the left, came on acutely 2 months ago, and is particularly aggravated by walking. As you talk to her more, she does not seem to be describing anterior hip or groin pain. The pain is more posterolateral in the gluteal area and not associated with any pain in the lumbar region. The pain does not radiate. She had X-rays of the hip taken a month ago, and these are normal with minimal osteoarthritis for age. She has a faint limp on the left leg when walking.

What do you do now?

Patients with the chief complaint of hip pain often refer to varying regions as their "hip." When approaching these patients, it is crucial to first specify the location of the pain. Often, the first question to ask is, "What do you mean by 'hip'?" Patients may distinguish regions such as their groin, thigh, buttocks, or low back as their "hip," and each region has different possible etiologies of pain (see Table 31.1). By clarifying what patients mean by "hip" and utilizing physical examination to evaluate for possible pathology, management can be better individualized.

Pain in the area of the hip can be initially categorized as predominantly anterior, lateral, or posterior when patients refer to a specific area of pain. Anterior pain, commonly indicated as groin pain by patients, often arises from the hip joint itself due to underlying osteoarthritis or labral pathology. Upper lumbar radiculopathies may also present with radiation in the groin and anterior thigh and should be considered. Additional possibilities include muscular injury to the hip flexors or hip adductors (which may be more common in younger athletes) or rarely a psoas hematoma in those on anti-coagulation medication. Osteitis pubis (inflammation of the pubic symphysis) and anterior pelvic or femoral stress fractures may also present

TABLE 31.1 **Differential Diagnosis of Hip Pain based on Region**

Anterior	Posterior	Lateral
· Hip osteoarthritis	· Referred pain from	· Greater trochanteric
· Labral pathology	spinal structures (L4/L5	pain syndrome (GTPS)
· Upper lumbar	and L5/S1 levels)	· Tendinopathy (most
radiculopathies	· Lumbar	commonly)
· Hip flexor/adductor	radiculopathy	· Bursitis (rare)
tendinopathy	· Facet arthropathy	Greater trochanteric
· Psoas hematoma	· Gluteal maximus or	avulsion fracture
· Osteitis pubis	hamstring tendonitis	· Lumbar
· Anterior pelvic or	· Inflammatory	radiculopathy
femoral stress	sacroiliitis	
fractures	· Sacral insufficiency	
· Inguinal hernia	fractures	
· Renal issues		
· Ovarian disorders		
· Septic arthritis		

with anterior hip/groin pain. Potential non-musculoskeletal etiologies include an inguinal hernia, renal issues, or an ovarian disorder.

Posterior "hip" pain has a wide differential. Spinal structures from the L4/L5 and L5/S1 levels, including discs, nerve roots, and facet joints, can all refer pain into the posterior gluteal area. Local muscular or tendinous issues, such as a strain of the gluteus maximus or hamstring tendonitis, and sacral or sacroiliac pathology can certainly result in posterior hip/pelvic pain. The latter would include inflammatory sacroiliitis or sacral insufficiency fractures which may be seen in endurance athletes or those with osteoporosis.

Lateral hip pain, which is the complaint of the patient presented above, is predominantly related to local structures at the greater trochanter, frequently subsumed as greater trochanteric pain syndrome (GTPS). GTPS is a general term used to describe disorders of the peri-trochanteric space, which can include insertional tendinopathies of the gluteus medius and/or minimus muscles or true trochanteric bursitis. Although lateral hip pain is frequently diagnosed as "greater trochanteric bursitis," true isolated bursitis at that location is actually rare; GTPS is generally a more appropriate term. Infrequently, lateral hip pain may result from either a problem with the femur itself, such as a greater trochanteric avulsion fracture after a fall, or a lumbar radiculopathy, particularly if associated with pain radiating down the lateral thigh and calf.

The prevalence of hip pain in the general population is estimated to be approximately 10% and increases with age. This number is difficult to interpret, as "hip" pain can obviously overlap with LBP and spinal or pelvic disorders, given the range of issues noted above. For younger patients, acute strains, tendinopathies, bone stress injuries, lumbar spine pathology, and hip joint labral tears are more common musculoskeletal etiologies of hip or pelvic pain. For older adults, hip osteoarthritis, GTPS, degenerative tendinopathies, and degenerative or discogenic lumbar spine disorders are most frequent.

A thorough history will help elucidate possible etiologies of a patient's hip pain. Standard questioning about onset, provoking/relieving activities, quality, radiation, severity, and timing can help clarify patients' symptoms. A history of trauma will affect diagnostic evaluation and can potentially evoke caution with certain exam maneuvers. Pain exacerbated by extension or flexion of the low back or associated radiating leg pain or paresthesia may indicate lumbar spine pathology. Transitional movements, such as when getting out of a car or changing from sitting to standing, may indicate intra-articular hip pathology or surrounding tendinopathies. Trouble with positioning the leg to put on shoes or socks is a frequent complaint with hip osteoarthritis. Stress fractures and musculotendinous strains generally have an acute onset and are worsened by weight-bearing. GTPS is frequently associated with walking or sleeping on the affected side and can be either gradual or acute in onset. It is always crucial to rule out red flag symptoms or other medical contributors. Fever may indicate possible infectious etiologies of pain such as a septic arthritis. As noted, the presence of a fracture is suggested by pain with weight-bearing. Pain at night, unplanned weight loss, and a history of prior cancer may indicate a possible tumor.

Physical examination for hip or pelvic area pain includes observation of gait and comprehensive evaluation of both the hip and spine. When assessing gait, observing a painful or antalgic gait is consistent with a range of possible problems in the hip or spine. A foot drop may suggest an L5 radiculopathy. The presence of a Trendelenburg gait or weakness of hip abduction upon single leg stance can be seen either with a lumbar radiculopathy (particularly L5) or with a greater trochanteric issue such as a tendinopathy. In a Trendelenburg gait, the contralateral hip falls toward the ground or the trunk leans to the ipsilateral side during the stance phase of gait (meaning that the right hip drops or the patient leans toward the left when standing only on the left leg during gait, for example). Palpation of relevant anatomic landmarks in the area of pain is helpful in identifying potentially affected structures. Assessing range of motion of the hip and for the presence of pain with hip flexion, abduction, and external rotation (FABER) and hip flexion, adduction, and internal rotation (FADIR) are essential parts of the examination, as abnormalities or pain may indicate hip joint pathology. For the spine exam, range of motion including flexion and extension within patient comfort should be observed for any significant restriction or reproduction of pain, and a basic neurological examination of the lower extremities should be performed.

Imaging studies can help sort through an appropriate differential diagnosis. Plain radiographs of the spine, hip, or pelvis may show correlative pathology. Magnetic resonance imaging (MRI) of the spine or pelvis can identify spine pathology, such as a disc herniation or spinal stenosis, and pelvic pathology, including soft tissue processes such as tendinitis, bursitis, strains, or muscular atrophy along with stress injuries to bone, sacroiliitis, joint inflammation, or tumors. Computed tomography, nuclear imaging, and ultrasound also may have select applications in assessing hip or pelvic pain. Clinicians have to be very careful to correlate the patient's presentation and physical examination with any imaging findings, however, as underlying imaging "abnormalities" are very common in asymptomatic populations. When assessing the association of hip pain with radiographic evidence of hip osteoarthritis in a study of over 4,000 patients, only 9% of hips in patients with frequent pain showed radiographic hip osteoarthritis, and only 24% of hips with radiographic hip osteoarthritis were frequently painful. Along with other spinal pathologies, disc degeneration is also common in asymptomatic individuals, ranging from 30% of 20-year-olds to 96% of 80-year-olds (see chapter 4). This emphasizes the importance of a comprehensive physical examination, as imaging and symptoms are not necessarily correlated. If a patient presents with anterior hip pain and has hip osteoarthritis on radiographs but has a normal hip exam, then the hip is unlikely to be the source of the patient's pain.

In approaching the patient presented above, we start with the knowledge that her pain is predominantly lateral. Despite the initial complaint of "hip" pain, there is actually a low concern for intra-articular hip pathology, given the lack of groin pain. This could be confirmed with a normal examination of the left hip. There is an antalgic gait with favoring of her right leg and pain on the left during left leg stance in the gait cycle. You do not observe any hip or foot drop. There is no limitation in lumbar spine range of motion. There is tenderness throughout the lateral hip with significant tenderness overlying the greater trochanter. Based on history and exam, you suspect the patient's pain is attributed to GTPS. GTPS typically presents in those >50 years old with a female-to-male ratio of approximately 4:1. It is estimated to have an annual incidence as high as 1.8 per 1000 adults. It presumably develops due to overload tendinopathy of the gluteus medius and minimus muscles which may result from maladaptive compensatory mechanisms due to prior foot, knee, or back problems.

There are limited data on the treatment of GTPS, in part likely related to the mixed pathologies that may present as GTPS. Conservative management is first-line with a focus on physical therapy. This should include isometric and closed chain exercises focusing on strengthening hip abductor musculature, functional retraining to reduce excess hip adduction with movements, and stretching of the iliotibial band. Aquatic therapy can be a good option for those with pain associated with walking. Recommendations for lifestyle modifications should include adjusting activities to reduce repetitive compression on the greater trochanter, such as sleeping side-lying or standing with legs crossed. The use of a cane or walking stick in the right arm during walking may reduce stress over the left greater trochanter, as well. Addressing weight, general exercise, and underlying health states, like smoking and diabetes, may be helpful in the long term.

Nonsteroidal anti-inflammatory drugs (NSAIDs)can be utilized to help with pain and assist with exercise therapies. Corticosteroid injections for GTPS may be more problematic than helpful. A randomized double-blind, placebo-controlled trial assessing efficacy of glucocorticoid injections to the greater trochanter for patients with GTPS showed that there was no greater efficacy of glucocorticoid injections compared to placebo. This data further suggest that GTPS is more related to tendinopathy, which would not be expected to respond as well to corticosteroid injection than the far less frequent true greater trochanteric bursitis. Studies on other tendinopathies have shown that corticosteroid injections are associated with worse long-term outcomes, and peripheral injections of corticosteroids can be associated with complications including adrenal suppression, reduced bone density, and tendon rupture. Surgery is rarely performed, as most patients respond to time and conservative care. For persistent symptoms and before considering interventional care like injections or surgery, it may be best to obtain imaging studies, such as MRI or ultrasound, to clarify the underlying pathology and adjust treatment as appropriate. Partial or complete tendon disruption with muscular atrophy represent relative contraindications to corticosteroid injections.

1. The complaint of "hip pain" can refer to a range of pathologies, many of which are not the actual hip joint. The location of pain in the hip, back, or pelvic region should guide differential diagnosis.
2. Physical examination is crucial for ascertaining the potential source of pain.
3. Imaging should not supersede physical examination, as imaging findings may not correlate with pain.
4. GTPS is a common etiology of lateral hip pain and is usually related to gluteal tendinopathy rather than true greater trochanteric bursitis.
5. GTPS generally responds to conservative management, including physical therapy and lifestyle modifications.

Further reading

1. Boyd M, Vijayaraghavan N, Karvelas K. Evidenced-based management of greater trochanteric pain syndrome. Curr Phys Med Rehabil Rep. 2020;8:313–321. https://doi.org/10.1007/s40141-020-00294-0.
2. Brinjikji W, Luetmer PH, Comstock B, et al. Systematic literature review of imaging features of spinal degeneration in asymptomatic populations. Am J Neuroradiol. 2015;36(4):811–816. https://doi.org/10.3174/ajnr.A4173.
3. Grimaldi A, Fearon A. Gluteal tendinopathy: integrating pathomechanics and clinical features in its management. J Orthopaed Sports Phys Ther. 2015;45(11):910–922. https://doi.org/10.2519/jospt.2015.5829.
4. Kim C, Nevitt MC, Niu J, et al. Association of hip pain with radiographic evidence of hip osteoarthritis: diagnostic test study. BMJ (Clinical research ed.). 2015;351:h5983. https://doi.org/10.1136/bmj.h5983.
5. Nissen MJ, Brulhart L, Faundez A, Finckh A, Courvoisier DS, Genevay S. (). Glucocorticoid injections for greater trochanteric pain syndrome: a randomised double-blind placebo-controlled (GLUTEAL) trial. Clin Rheumatol. 2019;38(3):647–655. https://doi.org/10.1007/s10067-018-4309-6.

32 "I Want to Stay in My Home.": An 87-Year-Old with Back Pain, Heart Failure, and Diabetes

Laura R. Lawson, Debra Kaye Weiner

An 87-year-old female presents with low back pain, present for several years. The pain radiates across her low back but not into her legs. It is bad when she stands for more than a few minutes. She tires easily. It is hard to prepare meals or care for her house. She is widowed and lives alone in a single-story home. She has had several near falls in her home, and she is afraid of falling. She can walk about 50 feet before she stops due to pain. Her medical history is notable for diabetes with nephropathy and peripheral neuropathy, congestive heart failure, and osteoporosis. Her medications include warfarin, metformin, lisinopril, trazodone, and furosemide. On exam, she is thin with a mild kyphoscoliosis. Her gait is unsteady. She has normal strength in her legs, loss of sensation to soft touch in a stocking-type distribution and loss of proprioception/vibration in her toes. X-rays show no fracture or spondylolisthesis but multilevel degenerative changes and mild kyphoscoliosis.

What do you do now?

First, we should acknowledge that chronic low back pain (LBP) is common, affecting 36–70% of older adults. Likewise, imaging showing disc degeneration is almost universal in patients over 80. It is important to educate the patient that her X-ray changes may not have any relation to her pain. We can be confident that dangerous causes of pain, like cancer or fracture, are extremely unlikely and should provide the patient with reassurance.

Though there are a multitude of physical conditions that can affect LBP, older adults are often plagued with other contributors to disability such as multimorbidity, polypharmacy, depression and anxiety, and frailty, each of which can be associated with increased pain interference (i.e. pain's interference with physical and/or emotional functioning and quality of life). The problem of chronic pain cannot be viewed in one dimension. All relevant biopsychosocial contributors should be addressed in the older adult with chronic pain to optimize treatment outcomes. It is critical that the provider educate patients about all treatment targets. By doing so, patients may be more willing to engage in the multifaceted approach required.

Frailty is a clinical state in which older adults are increasingly vulnerable to stressors (i.e. medical, environmental, and psychosocial) that lead to adverse health outcomes. This geriatric syndrome contributes to functional impairment that can manifest as weakness, slow walking speed, low physical activity and energy, tiredness, and weight loss. Frail older adults have increased mortality risk and are at risk of developing disability, dependence in activities of daily living, poor outcomes from medical procedures, and decreased quality of life. Our patient's chronic pain is a stressor that can directly contribute to frailty, and her tiredness could certainly be a symptom of this. There are many tools for evaluating frailty, but most are difficult to practically complete in the outpatient setting. The Clinical Frailty Scale, on the other hand, uses a simple visual scale with short descriptors to quickly categorize patients from "very fit" to "terminally ill" (see Figure 32.1). Once identified, frailty requires multifaceted treatment including optimizing medical conditions and nutrition, increasing physical activity and muscle mass, and mitigating the risks associated with frailty by optimizing home environment and social support. Physical therapy and nutrition referrals may be helpful to address aspects of frailty, and a comprehensive geriatrics

Clinical Frailty Scale*

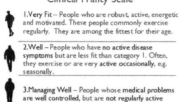

1. **Very Fit** – People who are robust, active, energetic and motivated. These people commonly exercise regularly. They are among the fittest for their age.

2. **Well** – People who have no active disease symptoms but are less fit than category 1. Often, they exercise or are very active occasionally, e.g. seasonally.

3. **Managing Well** – People whose medical problems are well controlled, but are not regularly active beyond routine walking.

4. **Vulnerable** – While not dependent on others for daily help, often symptoms limit activities. A common complaint is being "slowed up", and/or being tired during the day.

5. **Mildly Frail** – These people often have more evident slowing, and need help in high order IADLs (finances, transportation, heavy housework, medications). Typically, mild frailty progressively impairs shopping and walking outside alone, meal preparation and housework.

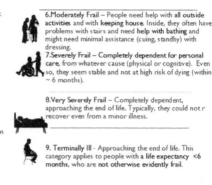

6. **Moderately Frail** – People need help with all outside activities and with keeping house. Inside, they often have problems with stairs and need help with bathing and might need minimal assistance (cuing, standby) with dressing.

7. **Severely Frail** – Completely dependent for personal care, from whatever cause (physical or cognitive). Even so, they seem stable and not at high risk of dying (within ~ 6 months).

8. **Very Severely Frail** – Completely dependent, approaching the end of life. Typically, they could not recover even from a minor illness.

9. **Terminally Ill** - Approaching the end of life. This category applies to people with a life expectancy <6 months, who are not otherwise evidently frail.

Scoring frailty in people with dementia

FIGURE 32.1. Clinical Frailty Scale.

evaluation should be considered to evaluate contributing factors and possible treatments.

Depression and anxiety are common but often unrecognized conditions in older adults. Instead of depressed mood, older adults with depression may present with somatic complaints such as fatigue, low energy, insomnia, or cognitive concerns. Some risk factors for depression in our patient include social isolation, chronic medical conditions, sedentary behavior, and chronic pain. The connection between pain and depression is not fully understood. However, we know that depression and pain are processed in shared brain regions including the insular cortex, prefrontal cortex, anterior cingulate, thalamus, hippocampus, and amygdala. This can lead to similar negative/maladaptive neuroplastic changes in the brain that can perpetuate these disease states. The Patient Health Questionnaire (PHQ) 2 is a well-validated depression screen. If positive, administration of the PHQ-9 is appropriate.

Generalized anxiety disorder (GAD) is the most common anxiety disorder in older adults. Common GAD risk factors are physical disability, stressful life changes, and previous mental health diagnoses. Additional risk factors that apply to our patient are social isolation and chronic medical conditions. Like depression, anxiety can present atypically in older adults with a preponderance of physical symptoms such as muscle tension, insomnia, and fatigue. Anxiety is processed in the same brain regions as pain and depression, perhaps accounting for the fact that anxiety is more common in patients with chronic pain than those without. All older adults with chronic pain should be screened for anxiety using the Generalized Anxiety Disorder 2-item (GAD-2) scale. If positive, the GAD-7 should be administered.

Treatment of anxiety and depression typically includes behavioral intervention such as interpersonal therapy and/or pharmacologic treatment, with selective serotonin reuptake inhibitors being first-line medication choices. If our patient is found to have anxiety or depression, treatment should be initiated and a referral for mental health services placed. This is likely to result in significant improvement in pain interference.

Because our patient is 87 years old, changes in her cognitive function should be considered. Conservatively, more than one-third of adults older than 85 have dementia, and chronic pain and dementia frequently coexist. Often older adults attribute their functional decline to chronic pain when, in fact, incipient dementia is the culprit. Our patient reports difficulty with preparing meals and caring for her home. Although there is insufficient evidence to recommend cognitive screening based on age alone, providers should have a low threshold for screening if there are any early signs of dementia (e.g. behavioral changes like apathy or social disinhibition, relinquishing hobbies, difficulty completing tasks, deficits in short-term memory, or subjective memory complaints). Screening can be easily completed in the office with the Mini-Cog©. This test requires the patient to recall a list of three words (i.e. banana, sunrise, chair) and draw a clock in a preprinted circle with the time indicating 10 past 11. One point is given for each word recalled, and two points for correct numbering and hand positioning on the clock. A score of less than 3 is considered a positive screen. A positive screen should be followed with more in-depth neuropsychological performance testing, identification of treatable contributors such as hypothyroidism and vitamin B12 deficiency, and consideration of specialist referral to geriatrics or neurology to guide behavioral and pharmacological treatment and planning for future care.

In addition to the psychosocial concerns related to our patient, falls are a prominent concern in the frail, older adult with chronic pain. Falls can cause significant injury and often can be prevented. Not all older patients will volunteer a fall history, so direct questioning and assessment of the patient's postural control should be routinely included as part of your assessment. Consider asking "Do you feel unsteady when standing or walking?" "Do you worry about falling?" "Have you fallen in the past year?" If the answer is "yes" to any of these questions, a functional evaluation should be done (these questions are in the Stopping Elderly Accidents, Deaths, and Injuries (STEADI) algorithm put out by the Centers for Disease Control). Despite our patient's unsteady gait and neuropathy, both of which are risk factors for falls, she does not report any recent falls, but she does report fear of falling and has a history of osteoporosis, putting her at risk for fall-related adverse events. Falls and fear of falling are associated with activity avoidance that, in itself, fosters greater pain and disablement.

Physical therapy should almost always be prescribed for the older adult with chronic LBP and can address improving balance (with or without an appropriate assistive device) and fitness, reducing fear of falling, and optimizing gait biomechanics. When joint and musculotendinous restrictions/tightness are present, physical therapists can instruct the patient in proper stretching techniques and perform manual therapy. Assistive device education is an important part of physical therapy. A wheeled walker can effectively reduce back pain by unloading the spine, especially in patients with kyphoscoliosis, as in our patient. Assistive devices also can be very helpful in reducing fear of falling and optimizing mobility, balance, and independence in daily functioning.

Before prescribing medication for pain, a thorough review of the patient's medical comorbidities and medications (including those that are nonprescription) should be conducted. This will afford identification of potential drug–drug and drug–disease interactions. We refer providers to Beers Criteria for Potentially Inappropriate Medications in Older Adults for a thorough list of important considerations (see Table 32.1 for common medications used in pain management that are included on the Beers list). In general, nonsteroidal anti-inflammatory drugs (NSAIDs) should be avoided in older adults because of potential renal, cardiac, and gastric toxicity and increased risk of bleeding in patients, such as ours, who are taking anticoagulants. Muscle relaxants, because of their significant anticholinergic potential and increased falls risk, also should be avoided in older adults. Acetaminophen is an overall safe first-line analgesic with a

TABLE 32.1 **Common Medications used to Treat Pain. Excerpt from the American Geriatrics Society Beers Criteria® for Potentially Inappropriate Medication Use in Older Adults**

Medication	Patient Factors That Increase Risk	Concern
Opioids	Fall risk, on concurrent gabapentinoids or benzodiazepines	Unsteady gait, syncope, sedation, respiratory depression, death, overdose
Tramadol	Renal impairment	SIADH, CNS adverse effects
Gabapentinoids (i.e. Gabapentin, Pregabalin)	Renal impairment, concurrent opioid use	CNS adverse effects, sedation, respiratory depression, death
Muscle relaxants (i.e. cyclobenzaprine, methocarbamol)		Anticholinergic effects, questionably efficacy at doses tolerated in older patients
NSAIDs	Heart failure, ulcer history, creatinine clearance <30 mL/min	GI bleed, kidney injury, increased blood pressure, worsening heart failure
COX-2 Inhibitors	Heart failure, creatinine clearance <30 mL/min	Worsening heart failure, worsening renal function in chronic kidney disease

suggested maximum dose of 3000 mg (less in patients with liver dysfunction). Topical lidocaine, menthol, and capsaicin are all safe and generally well-tolerated. Providers should be aware that older adults have increased pharmacodynamic sensitivity to opioids, and if such a medication is felt to be indicated to alleviate refractory pain-related suffering, 50% of the typical starting dose should be utilized. Additionally, informed consent should include education of opioid-associated risks in older adults over and above those that can be experienced by patients of any age (e.g. delirium, falls, and hip fracture).

For the patient presented here, we should let her know that there is no evidence of one specific, reversible cause of her pain, such as injury.

Although we want to improve her pain, successful pain treatment is not just a reduction in pain severity. We should also explore other goals, such as improving physical function, improving safety, maintaining independence in the home, and preventing frailty. To do this, we must address not only her pain but also her comorbid conditions, medications, and mobility.

Her neuropathy and fear of falling clearly suggest she is a fall risk. We should refer her to physical therapy to assess gait and stability and suggest a possible assistive device. A physical therapist can also develop a home exercise program for range of motion, stretching, and strengthening to address chronic pain. Physical therapy and/or occupational therapy could review her home environment to determine appropriate alterations and durable medical equipment that could be helpful. Her medications should be reevaluated on a regular basis, regardless of chronicity. Patients are continuously changing with age and their medications should, too. Our patient is on furosemide and trazodone, both of which can cause dehydration and orthostasis. Orthostatic vital signs can be checked and a dose reduction considered, if positive. A noticeable omission from her medication list is treatment for osteoporosis. Her past bone mineral density testing should be reviewed to determine if treatment or further testing is needed.

Her chronic pain and social isolation put her at risk for depression and anxiety, and she should be screened for both. We should educate her that poor mood can contribute to worsening or uncontrolled pain. It is important that she understand that physical and mental health are connected and both need to be addressed for her to feel her best.

Pharmacological treatment with use of acetaminophen or topical preparations can be considered as adjuncts to the interventions above.

KEY POINTS

1. Radiographic evidence of degenerative disc disease is common and nonspecific in older adults; it is as likely to be present in those with and without pain.
2. Physical therapy is an important intervention that can address many of the physical factors that contribute to pain or develop due to pain.

3. Treatment of chronic low back pain requires comprehensive assessment to identify the multiple biopsychosocial treatment targets that are typically present in older adults, such as frailty, depression, anxiety, and cognitive decline.
4. Treatment of older adults with chronic pain should focus not only on pain reduction but improving function and maintaining independence.

Further reading

1. 2019 American Geriatrics Society Beers Criteria® Update Expert Panel. American Geriatrics Society 2019 updated AGS Beers Criteria® for potentially inappropriate medication use in older adults. J Am Geriatr Soc. 2019;67(4):674–694. doi:10.1111/jgs.15767.
2. Centers for Disease Control. STEADI algorithm for fall risk screening, assessment, and intervention among community-dwelling adults 65 years and older. 2019. Accessed 12-23-2021. https://www.cdc.gov/steadi/pdf/STEADI-Algorithm-508.pdf.
3. Weiner DK. Deconstructing chronic low back pain in the older adult: shifting the paradigm from the spine to the person. Pain Medicine. 2015;16(5):881–885. https://doi.org/10.1111/pme.12759.
4. Weiner DK, Marcum Z, Rodriguez E. Deconstructing chronic low back pain in older adults: summary recommendations. Pain Medicine. 2016;17(12):2238–2246. https://doi.org/10.1093/pm/pnw267.

33 "I Need to Exercise to Lose Weight, but My Back Hurts.": Low Back Pain with a BMI of 47

Alex Watson, Christopher J. Standaert

You see a 66 year-old-patient with concerns about her weight. She has a BMI of 47 and has gained about 80 lbs. over the last 10–15 years. She just retired and was hoping to work on her health in general. As she tried to walk more, she started getting pain in her low back. This has become a limiting factor in how far she can walk. She does not have leg pain or numbness or other neurologic change. She had some radiographs done showing a mild degenerative scoliosis with multilevel degenerative change and faint spondylolistheses at L3/L4 and L4/L5. There is no instability on flexion/extension films. She is trying to watch her diet but knows she needs to exercise more to lose weight.

What do you do now?

This patient presents with an expressed desire to improve her health but has significant barriers revolving around her low back and her obesity. To help improve her current state, these have to be addressed concurrently. From a spine perspective, she has degenerative issues on imaging, which are not uncommon for her age. The spondylolistheses and scoliosis each present distinct challenges, but exercise, weight loss, and general good health behaviors are central to the management of both (see chapters 9 and 10 for a discussion of these diagnoses). Obesity clearly complicates this whole scenario, and addressing the obesity requires interdisciplinary care as the sequelae of metabolic disease span nearly all body systems. As body mass index (BMI) increases, the musculoskeletal impacts and association with low back pain (LBP) are significant. This patient needs to understand that treating her back will require an integrated approach to addressing her overall health, as isolated approaches to try to improve her LBP long-term are likely to be ineffective.

Already one of the most common and costliest health conditions, the prevalence of LBP is even higher in those with obesity. This population has higher rates of chronic pain in general—approximately 33% vs. 10% in the average population. This is at least partially related to adipose tissue secreting pro-inflammatory cytokines. Many of the environmental/behavioral contributors to obesity such as the "standard American diet" and sedentary behavior are associated with greater pain sensitivity as well. Obstructive sleep apnea, a common obesity-associated disease, is also highly associated with chronic pain; the disordered sleep then contributes to further weight gain by worsening insulin resistance and elevations in the "hunger hormone" ghrelin which stimulates appetite further. Leptin resistance, another phenomenon seen in patients with obesity, has also been associated with joint pain and erosion. During painful episodes, individuals often report eating more and loss of control of eating behaviors. Even when controlling for negative mood and BMI, acute pain/ pain level precipitates increased consumption of sweet foods and higher total calories. Sedentary behavior also becomes self-sustaining, as the phenomenon of kinesiophobia, an irrational and exaggerated fear response to movement, leads to reduced activity out of concern for worsening pain. Often, the level of functional disability is not fully explained by the severity of acute/chronic LBP.

Obesity-related diseases, such as diabetes, hypertension, and hyperlipidemia, further complicate an already impaired health state and present additional barriers to exercise and other forms of care. Although those with obesity are prone to the same spinal disorders as individuals with normal weight, there is reason to believe that obesity may contribute to the development of degenerative issues, like degenerative scoliosis and spondylolisthesis (as seen in the patient presented), and obesity is associated with worse outcomes for treatment of these conditions. Obesity also clearly increases the risk of specific cancers, and the combination of obesity and sarcopenia may have a particularly negative effect on bone health. All of these need to be considered when evaluating an individual with obesity and LBP.

During the initial patient assessment, practitioners must be mindful of the many limitations to providing good care for patients with obesity, such as limited time for motivational interviewing, fear of offending patients with poor word choices, and lack of knowledge/comfort recommending weight loss treatments. Despite this, many patients with obesity report wanting their doctor to initiate the conversation about weight management. Begin using a standard approach to motivational interviewing by asking permission to address the patient's weight, as it may be related to his or her back pain. In these conversations, patients often prefer clinicians use terms like "weight" or "BMI" instead of "obesity," "size," or "fatness." Also, avoid any implication of blame as obesity is multifactorial, and a judgmental tone will limit the productivity of the conversation.

All patients with LBP need an examination of gait, spinal and hip motion, and lower extremity strength, sensation, and reflexes. For patients with obesity, the physical assessment should include measuring height, weight with BMI calculations, waist and neck circumference, serum fasting glucose, and a lipid profile. Reviewing these results with patients may help increase motivation for interventions by illustrating the scope of metabolic disease, and these data also provide a baseline for tracking progress. Weight alone, for example, is a poor metric to monitor, as increases in lean muscle mass may obscure progress in losing fat mass. Include a basic safety screening to determine risk of cardiac disease which may prompt additional targeted assessments.

With these considerations in mind, clinical discussions should include options for weight loss, reiterating the direct and indirect benefits to the patient's LBP. Traditionally, lifestyle interventions are recommended as the first-line treatment for weight loss, but in the context of obesity-related complications such as musculoskeletal pain, practitioners should discuss a multimodal approach with lifestyle interventions and pharmacologic support. Exercise is a necessary component of mitigating LBP in patients with obesity (see Figure 33.1). Clarifying the mechanism of the onset of disability may allow providers to tailor treatments by incrementally exposing the patient to feared movements with supervision. Gradually this will reduce apprehension, improve function, and demonstrate tolerance to brief, acute increases in inflammation seen during bouts of exercise. Research on multiple exercise strategies supports the efficacy of the common adage "the best form of exercise is the kind that you will do."

Ultimately, all exercise regimens benefit LBP, but aquatic therapy is a uniquely beneficial modality in those with obesity. Offloading axial forces and the effect of water immersion on pain perception may acutely reduce LBP during the exercise session. Aquatic exercise also offers a favorable safety

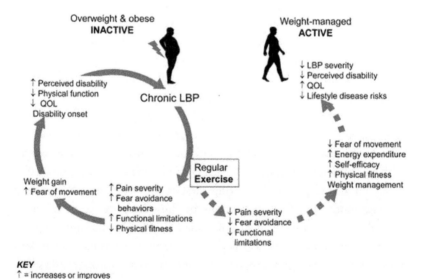

FIGURE 33.1. Benefits of exercise for low back pain in overweight and obesity.

From: Wasser JG, et al. Exercise benefits for chronic low back pain in overweight and obese individuals. PM&R. 2017;9(2):181–192.

profile as the buoyancy reduces the risk of joint injury, allowing individuals with obesity to exercise more vigorously than may be possible on land. Because of thermo-conductive effects, aquatic exercise also reduces heat stress/discomfort, which may improve adherence to the exercise program.

Aquatic-based physical therapy is available in many areas, and most public or membership-based swimming pools offer group aquatic fitness classes for added social benefit. In one study of women with obesity and LBP, a twice weekly aquatic exercise program of 60 minutes per session significantly improved myriad aspects of disability including pain intensity and the impact on personal care, sitting, standing, employment, and overall disability. Although the perceived exertion may be less if the patient is more comfortable in water, weight loss remains significant with additional improvements in strength, endurance, and pain symptoms.

For those without access to aquatic therapy, total body resistance training and yoga/Pilates programs are other appropriate options for exercise. Resistance/weight training can increase lean muscle mass and may offer subsequent additional benefits of improved insulin sensitivity, increased bone density, and resilience to falls.

Bariatric surgery may be warranted for individuals with obesity who either have multiple metabolic comorbidities or have a BMI >35 despite prior weight loss. Often, patients with LBP report improvements in pain frequency, severity, and disability following bariatric surgery. However, these procedures should not be considered an intervention to treat pain. Instead, they help restore healthy metabolic and biomechanical function, and, with these changes, pain symptoms may improve. For patients with obesity and clear structural spinal abnormalities for which surgery is indicated, bariatric surgery may reduce surgical risk and improve outcomes of subsequent spinal procedures.

Applying this discussion to the patient presented above, she would qualify for all possible counseling, pharmacology, and surgical interventions for weight loss given her BMI of 47. If she were open to both medical and surgical options, her best plan would be a full multimodal diet, exercise, and pharmacologic approach with a bariatric surgery consultation. Prior to recommending an exercise regimen, an assessment of tolerance may help guide the recommendations—as her pain is limiting, aquatic therapy would be a better setting than land-based fitness equipment. If her available time is not restrictive, then complementing multiple training styles, such as resistance training and aquatic therapy, as part of physical therapy could provide for faster gains in strength and physical resilience while effectively decreasing pain and disability. Clinicians should address mood disorders early and in a straightforward manner or have the patient follow-up with a psychiatrist/psychologist as needed. If the patient's history includes symptoms suggestive of disordered sleeping, she should be referred to a sleep specialist. As she progresses through her multimodal program, she should then gradually increase her walking distance as tolerated for additional potential benefit.

This pre-habilitation prior to potential bariatric surgery may also benefit the patient's recovery and outcomes from surgery, if applicable. By incorporating a surgical consultation early, the patient can begin the months-long process of qualifying for bariatric surgery, often requiring a period of weight loss/maintenance prior to surgery. When presenting this intervention, one must be careful to stress that the bariatric surgery itself will not directly improve pain but allow for accelerated weight loss and improvements in other markers of health. Often, this is suggested after trials of nutritional, exercise, and pharmacotherapy interventions.

KEY POINTS

1. Obesity and its comorbidities are associated with increased pain sensitivity.
2. For patients with obesity and low back pain without structural spinal pathology, addressing obesity with a multimodal approach is the best way to treat pain.
3. Word choice matters in motivational interviewing. Start by asking for permission to discuss the patient's weight, as it is likely contributing to their pain.
4. The best choice of exercise is something the patient enjoys and will consistently perform. Given multiple choices, aquatic therapy has unique benefits for patients with obesity.
5. Addressing comorbidities, like sleep and mood disorders, will likely increase the efficacy of other interventions.

Further reading

1. Shiri R, Karppinen J, Leino-Arjas P, Solovieva S, Viikari-Juntura E. The association between obesity and low back pain: a meta-analysis. Am J Epidemiol. 2010;171(2):135–154.
2. Bessell E, Markovic TP, Fuller NR. How to provide a structured clinical assessment of a patient with overweight or obesity. Diabetes Obes Metab. 2021;23(S1):36–49.
3. Becker BE. Aquatic therapy: scientific foundations and clinical rehabilitation applications. PM&R. 2009;1(9):859–872.
4. Wasser JG, Vasilopoulos T, Zdziarski LA, Vincent HK. Exercise benefits for chronic low back pain in overweight and obese individuals. PM&R. 2017;9(2):181–192.
5. Stefanova I, Currie AC, Newton RC, Albon L, Slater G, Hawkins W, Pring C. A meta-analysis of the impact of bariatric surgery on back pain. Obes Surg. 2020;30(8):3201–3207.

34 "I Have Tried Everything for My Back Pain!": What to Do When There Is Nothing Left to Do

Christopher J. Standaert

You have seen your 46-year-old patient multiple times for low back pain over the past few years. Over the counter medication, walking for exercise, and physical therapy (PT) were unhelpful. You obtained X-rays and referred them to a surgeon. After a magnetic resonance imaging (MRI) study was performed, the surgeon said surgery would not help them. The patient then went to a pain management specialist. An unspecified injection in their back only helped for 2 days. They declined an antidepressant medication and referral to a psychologist, noting "the pain is not in my head." Chiropractic care only helped for a few hours after each visit, so they stopped going. Reports of the X-rays and MRI describe "degenerative disc disease" but nothing else that seems significant. Your patient wonders about quitting their job, has gained 20 lbs. over a few years, is not sleeping well, and is irritable at home. Frustrated, they look at you and exclaim, "I have tried everything!"

What do you do now?

About 30% of adults in the United States experience chronic LBP, and about half of those note the pain has lasted for 5 years or longer. LBP is more common with increasing age, more common in women than in men, highest for non-Hispanic White people and lowest for non-Hispanic Asians with Black and Hispanic populations falling somewhere between those two. It is more common in those living below the federal poverty level than in those with family incomes above that level. On the whole, chronic LBP is best approached as a biopsychosocial problem rather than a strictly anatomic issue, and clinicians need to understand the reality that there is no medication proven to be highly effective in treating chronic LBP and that there are no surgical or interventional procedures that have been shown to reliably provide long-term relief of chronic LBP. This all correlates with data indicating that, as of 2016, more money was spent in the care of LBP and neck pain in the United States than on any other medical condition.

With this background, it is understandable that many patients are frustrated with both their pain and their care, not infrequently noting that they feel as though they "have tried everything."

This is a challenging position for a clinician. Part of this challenge lies in transitioning the patient to an understanding that treating chronic LBP is more about managing their situation and improving their overall health and quality of life rather than "fixing" their pain. The ultimate goal of treatment is really behavioral change. To achieve this, there is also a responsibility on the clinician to ensure that an appropriate medical evaluation, psychosocial history, and exploration of barriers related to belief structures and social factors have actually been performed and that any issues identified have been addressed correctly. Patients also frequently do not understand the role of physical therapy, the language in MRI reports, the role of specific medications, injections, or surgery; or the relationship between emotional state, life circumstances, stress, physical activity, sleep, and pain. Helping them put these in context can be dramatically beneficial. If there is a persistent belief that they "have a disease," that their spine "is falling apart," or that there is some magical pill, shot, or surgery that will "fix" them, then their pain and limitations will be very difficult to manage.

From a medical standpoint, it is helpful to go back through their history and medical workup. Clearly, screening for red flag conditions, specifically tumor and infection, are important in those with chronic recalcitrant LBP.

These are discussed in chapters 14 and 15, but a history of cancer, immunosuppression, intravenous drug use, or constitutional symptoms, like unexplained weight loss, should prompt further evaluation. Conditions that can present with LBP but do not routinely appear on spine imaging include seronegative spondyloarthropathies (chapter 30) and intra- abdominal disorders. The latter can include conditions like esophagitis or pancreatitis, which can cause thoracic or upper lumbar pain, endometriosis or ovarian cysts, an aortic process (typically a more acute concern), renal issues/nephrolithiasis, cholecystitis, or other conditions that may affect the peritoneum or retroperitoneal space. These should be considered when the patient does not relate any real response to mechanical measures directed toward their spine. Musculoskeletal problems in the pelvis may also manifest as LBP. Examples to consider are conditions like greater trochanteric pain syndrome (chapter 31), a sacral or pubic ramus fracture, hip osteoarthritis, or musculotendinous injuries (such as gluteus maximus or medius strains, or hamstring tendinopathy). Abdominal imaging can help in the evaluation of possible intra-abdominal or pelvic pathology, pelvic/hip radiographs can show osteoarthritis or similar bone/ joint problems, a pelvic MRI can identify a musculotendinous injury or avascular necrosis (among other orthopedic conditions), and laboratory studies can be useful in the diagnosis of rheumatologic, infectious, or other medical conditions. Occasionally, referral to a gynecologist, gastroenterologist, or other medical specialist may be appropriate if there is concern for a non-spinal process.

MRIs present a number of issues. MRI readings vary substantially between radiologists, and relevant findings may be difficult to discern from a long list of age-appropriate findings. In those with radicular symptoms, findings of a disc extrusion or sequestration may be particularly important to identify. Far lateral disc herniations (chapter 6) are often suboptimally visualized and may be frequently mistaken clinically for a hip process. A spondylolisthesis may be missed if plain radiographs are not obtained in the standing position. It is important that all spine images be reread by a spine provider and/or radiologist with a thorough description of the patient's clinical presentation in mind. Sometimes the right test has been performed but not interpreted correctly, and sometimes the right test has not yet been done. Given the high rate of "abnormalities" on MRIs in asymptomatic people (chapter 4), it is critical to correlate the imaging to the clinical presentation.

The language used in reports of spine MRIs or other imaging is also problematic and may be associated with unintended iatrogenic harm. Words like "rupture," "degeneration," "severe," and "disease" can be frightening for patients. Studies have consistently shown that, compared to patients who have their inconsequential MRI findings described as "age-appropriate" in some form, those who receive detailed radiology reports tend to have worse outcomes and a lesser sense of well-being. Patients with chronic LBP often cannot put the language of imaging reports into context. Those with chronic pain also tend to see any described "abnormality" as validation that their ongoing pain is "real" and not "in their head." These perceptions can then be associated with fear of further injury, a belief that their problem can be "fixed" (as it is clearly visible on the MRI), or that they are destined to live in a fragile state with only further problems arising from their spine. All of these disempower the patient from improving their own situation. Addressing poor sleep, lack of exercise, fear, anxiety, diet, deconditioning, unnecessary (if not harmful) medications, and concurrent medical conditions are all examples of ways to improve health, quality of life, and pain that are independent from the findings on an MRI.

Understanding the role of physical therapy and other treatment approaches is critical. Many patients will say that physical therapy did not help their pain or that it was otherwise ineffective. Reasons for this can vary, but many patients mistakenly believe that PT is intended to cure their pain. When this does not happen within a few visits, they feel that "PT did not work." In some acute settings, PT can help with pain. In the more chronic state, PT is really intended to help patients understand that they can move without causing harm and to help them engage in an appropriate exercise program outside of PT. Using an active, encouraging, exercise-based approach, patients should be taught how their body and spine work, where they may be weak or tight, and how to exercise to compensate for any problems they may have. This should be done in a manner that fosters an appropriate long-term exercise program intended to help them feel better, function better, and be less susceptible to injury. PT is more of a gateway to a healthier way of living than it is an endpoint in "curing" the pain. The most important component of therapeutic exercise for chronic LBP is actually instilling the belief that improvement is possible. In all cases of chronic pain, having a goal to obtain (other than solely elimination of pain, which is both unrealistic and a barrier to improvement in other ways) is critical and helps the patient "buy in." Establishing a goal like walking a mile, lifting a child, playing golf, mowing a lawn, playing piano, or running a marathon is central to improvement in PT. In general, if someone does not know where they want to go, it is very hard to help them get there.

Medications and surgery are similar conceptually. Medications can be helpful for specific purposes, such as acute pain relief, sleep induction, treatment of anxiety or depression, or reduction of inflammation. There is no medication that has been shown to be highly effective in the long-term relief of pain in those with chronic LBP. Using medication in an attempt to "eliminate" pain is both unsuccessful and generally detrimental. Using medication to address specific aspects of a patient's pain state and to foster independent function and self-care may be more helpful. Similarly, surgery is generally not effective for the treatment of isolated axial LBP. Surgery is far more successful in the treatment of radicular pain in settings like a disc herniation or spinal stenosis. Patients should not be given the perception that, if all else fails, there is a surgery that will "fix" their LBP. Like imaging, this creates the belief that pain is purely structural and that the solution is out of their own control.

A final consideration in a patient like the one presented here is to really understand their social and psychological existence, their childhood, their coping methods, and their approach to challenges and trauma. Adverse childhood experiences, trauma, injustice, marginalization, discrimination, and abuse all negatively impact outcomes and function in the setting of LBP. They may also create distrust in the care system or result in a very protective approach to avoiding further harm. In many contexts, "exercise" is a luxury. Those struggling more with basic economic or psychological survival may find the concept of exercise, as espoused by many in the fitness world, as completely foreign or unobtainable. Some may lack the financial resources, time, transportation, or physical access to spaces that facilitate exercise. Some may also have those in their life that do not support or fundamentally obstruct the pursuit of exercise or independent health. Living in an unsafe, emotionally, or physically abusive or isolated setting can create these circumstances. When "exercise" is either inaccessible or unhelpful conceptually, it may be better to reframe the discussion around "movement" and "activity."

Coping mechanisms can go different ways with chronic LBP. Those who tend to be more passive and retreat due to fear do poorly and need to be encouraged to believe that they can and will be OK if they move. Those who tend to believe that they can outwork any obstacle also tend to do poorly as healing, improving physical performance, and modifying physical skills takes time and patience. It is often helpful to explain to these individuals that it is the tortoise that wins the race, not the hare. People simply cannot outwork biology but, instead, need to be methodical in how they approach exercise and recovery. Failure to do so often results in lack of progress, recurrent pain, and frustration.

So what can one do to help the patient described above? First, listen to their story. As it is clear by now that there is no readily apparent solution to their LBP, this will take some time. This discussion should include their experience of LBP, how they have perceived attempts at treatment, what they might be afraid of or wish could be done, what their prior experience with pain and trauma has been, and how their life has been impacted by their pain. Motivational interviewing skills can be helpful. Next, providers should comprehensively run through diagnostic possibilities, including consideration of inflammatory or non-spinal sources of pain, and go through existing imaging and other medical evaluation to ensure that nothing has been missed and that the correct studies have been done. A thorough physical examination should be done with the same diagnostic considerations in mind. In this process, providers need to be exploring potential goals and barriers to improvement. The patient will need an explanation of the significance or lack thereof of any findings on imaging. Further medical evaluation obtained should similarly be explained. The patient will also need an explanation as to the purpose of physical therapy, medications, or other treatment options considered. All treatment needs to be based on what was learned from the above.

Finally, a discussion about goals, the use of treatment approaches as tools to achieve those goals, specific barriers that are apparent, a motivational conversation about the need to invest in improving, and a promise not to abandon the patient along the way is needed. If the patient was happy with their current state, they would not be talking to you. Sometimes that acknowledgment alone is the place to start. They are not sleeping well, have gained weight, and are irritable with those they care about. That all has to change. Sleep, exercise, diet, social engagement, and goals/passions are fundamental human needs. Treatment from here focuses on those rather than pain relief, with the understanding that the goal is to improve their life. Redirected physical therapy aimed at mobility, conditioning, and achieving a meaningful goal; assistance with sleep hygiene; a dietician; a health coach, if available; and maybe a psychology referral may all be helpful here. In this process, the patient must feel as though they have been heard. Guiding them to a better space will take time, and they should be given routine follow-up appointments on a monthly basis for a while to help them through this.

KEY POINTS

1. No one has actually done "everything."
2. A thorough medical evaluation includes exploration of alternative diagnoses and obtaining appropriate diagnostic studies, as well as ensuring that existing studies have been interpreted correctly.
3. Often, patients who have not benefited from physical therapy have incorrectly expected that the treatment was intended to "fix" their pain rather than engage them in rehabilitation.
4. It is critical to understand the patient's psychological experience with pain and trauma, their beliefs, and their goals.
5. Sleep, exercise, diet, social engagement, and goal directed behaviors form the fundamental goals of care.

Further reading
1. Brinjikji W, Luetmer PH, Comstock B, et al. Systematic literature review of imaging features of spinal degeneration in asymptomatic populations. Am J Neuroradiol. 2015 Apr;36(4):811–816. doi: 10.3174/ajnr.A4173. Epub 2014 Nov 27.
2. Medina-Mirapeix F, Escolar-Reina P, Gascón-Cánovas JJ, Montilla-Herrador J, Collins SM. Personal characteristics influencing patients' adherence to home exercise during chronic pain: a qualitative study. J Rehabil Med. 2009 Apr;41(5):347–352.

3. Sharma S, Traeger AC, Reed B, et al. Clinician and patient beliefs about diagnostic imaging for low back pain: a systematic qualitative evidence synthesis. BMJ Open. 2020 Aug 23;10(8):e037820.
4. Steiger F, Wirth B, de Bruin ED, Mannion AF. Is a positive clinical outcome after exercise therapy for chronic non-specific low back pain contingent upon a corresponding improvement in the targeted aspect(s) of performance? A systematic review. Eur Spine J. 2012 Apr;21(4):575–598.

Index

For the benefit of digital users, indexed terms that span two pages (e.g., 52–53) may, on occasion, appear on only one of those pages.

Tables and figures are indicated by an italic *t* and *f* following the page number.

braces
  benefits/limitations of, 78
  children/adolescents, 216–17
  focal/ongoing back pain, 28
  progressive scoliosis, 91
  TLSO, 118
  vertebral compression fracture, 100–1
breast cancer, 98–100
breastfeeding, 251, 254–55
brick column analogy, 78–79
brucellosis, 128
burst fracture
  case study, 113
  characterization, 114–16, 115f
  differential diagnosis, 114, 119
  epidemiology, 115–16
  imaging, 116–17, 117f, 118
  neurological evaluation, 116, 118
  outcomes, 118–19
  physical examination, 116, 118
  referrals, 118
  surgery, 116, 118
  treatment, 116, 118

cancer
  cauda equina syndrome and, 122–
    23, 124–25
  chemotherapy/radiation therapy, 125
  differential diagnosis, 57–58, 243, 247
  metastases, imaging, 98–100
  myelopathy and, 123
  new onset pain, 121–26
  obesity in etiology of, 285
  TNF inhibitors contraindicated, 263
canes, 91
capsaicin, 278–79
catastrophizing, 145, 151, 167–68, 170
cauda equina syndrome
  anatomy, 136
  cancer and, 122–23, 124–25
  case study, 135
  cauda equina compression, 88, 136, 140
  clinical presentation, 136, 139–40
  confirmation of diagnosis, 137–38

consultation, 138–39
corticosteroids, 139
differential diagnosis, 42, 48–49,
  88, 243
first responder actions, 140
imaging, 137, 138f, 140, 247
lumbar spinal stenosis and, 57–58
neurological exam, 137, 138–39, 140
office vs. ER evaluation, 136
physical examination, 116
post-discectomy, 176–77
surgery, 139, 246
Charcot spine
  characterization, 224–25, 225f, 229
  differential diagnosis, 223, 224–25
  imaging, 225f, 225, 227f, 227
  recurrence, 227–28
  risk factors, 226
  surgery, 227–28
chest expansion test, 261
children/adolescents
  case study, 209–10
  differential diagnosis, 211–12
  epidemiology, 211, 218
  etiologies, 212
  imaging, 215–16, 217–18
  pars fracture defect, 209–18, 213f,
    215f, 216f
  physical examination, 214–15
  return to play, 218
  risk factors, 211
  treatment, 216–17, 218
chiropractic, 91, 161, 162
cholecystitis, 292–93
chronic low back pain
  case study, 291
  characterization, 292, 297
  coping mechanisms, 296, 297
  history taking/evaluation, 292–93, 295–
    96, 297
  imaging, 293–94
  imaging/language of imaging, 293–94
  management, 294–96
  treatment, 292, 296–97

fear-avoidant beliefs, 163
imaging, 160
litigation impacts, 161
management, 161–62
medications, 161, 162
physical examination, 159, 164
prognosis, 160–61, 162–63
psychosocial risk factor screening,
163, 164
referrals, 163
multiple sclerosis, 263
muscle aging effects, 195–96
muscle relaxants
acute low back pain, 10
depression/anxiety, 147
focal/ongoing back pain, 28
motor vehicle collision, 161
older adults, 279t
radiating leg pain, 42–43
tennis-related pain, 198–99
muscle strain differential diagnosis, 88
myeloma, 125
myelopathy, 61–62, 123

neoplasms. *See* cancer
nephrolithiasis, 51, 292–93
neuropathic pain, 223, 224, 228
neuropathic spinal arthropathy. *See*
Charcot spine
new onset pain
case study, 121
differential diagnosis, 229
ER referral, 124–25, 126
etiologies, 223–24
history taking/evaluation, 122–23, 126
imaging, 123
lesion evaluation, 123–24
multidisciplinary approach to, 126
neuropathic, 223, 224, 228
nonsurgical management, 125
physical examination, 123
red flag conditions, 122–23, 126
spinal metastases, 122

surgery, 124–25
TLICS score in management, 124, 126
nortriptyline, 255
NSAIDs
acute low back pain, 10
axial spondyloarthritis, 262–63
children/adolescents, 216–17
degenerative spondylolisthesis, 80
fibromyalgia, 154–55
focal/ongoing back pain, 23
hip pathology, 270
motor vehicle collision, 161, 162
older adults, 278–79, 279t
postoperative pain, 180
postpartum pain, 252
progressive scoliosis, 89–90
radiating leg pain, 42–43, 44
running-related injuries, 189
tennis-related pain, 198–99
vertebral compression fracture, 100

obesity
bariatric surgery, 287
case study, 283
characterization, 284–85, 288
clinical presentation, 284
golf pain, 202
patient assessment, 285
recurrent low back pain, 17
weight loss management, 285–87,
286f, 288
occiput to wall test, 261
older adults
case study, 273–74
cognitive function testing, 277
depression/anxiety in, 276–77, 280
falls in, 277–78, 280
frailty in, 275–76, 276f
lower back pain in, 275, 280
medications, 278–79, 279t
physical therapy, 278, 280
radiculitis/radiculopathy in, 62
treatment, 279–80, 281

clinical presentation, 243
differential diagnosis, 243, 244t,
    247, 251
imaging, 243–45, 247
low back/pelvic pain in, 242–43, 247
medications, 246
physical examination, 243, 247
postpartum pain, 249–54
treatment, 245–46, 247
progressive scoliosis. *See also* scoliosis
body weight, 91–92, 93
case study, 85–86
Cobb angle, 87, 88f, 89, 93
curve progression, 89
differential diagnosis, 87, 88
epidemiology, 87
history taking/evaluation, 87–88
imaging, 88f, 89, 90f, 92–93
management, 89–93
medications, 89–90
monitoring, 92
occupational therapy, 92–93
physical examination, 89
physical therapy, 90–91, 92–93
sagittal imbalance, 89, 90f
surgery, 92
PROMIS scale, 92
Promoting Amputee Life Skills, 238
prostate cancer, 98–100
prosthesis. *See* people with limb loss
proximal hamstring tendinopathy, 184
psoas hemorrhage, 51
PTSD
fibromyalgia and, 151, 152
motor vehicle collision, 160–61
people with limb loss, 233–34, 238, 239
PWLL. *See* people with limb loss

quadriceps weakness, 237

radiating leg pain. *See also* disc herniation
case study, 39
differential diagnosis, 251

disc anatomy, 40, 41f
history taking/evaluation, 41–42, 44, 45
imaging, 42, 44
medications, 42–43, 44
outcome predictors, 45
pathophysiology, 40, 45
surgery, 43–44
terminology, 40
treatment, 42–44, 45
radiculitis/radiculopathy
chronic low back pain, 295
defined, 40
differential diagnosis, 2, 51, 57, 71–72,
    82, 87, 89, 175, 176t, 214, 244t, 266t
disc extrusions/sequestrations,
    34, 293–94
electrodiagnostic testing, 71–72
epidural steroid injections, 26, 43,
    44, 246
hip pathology, 266t, 267, 268
imaging, 42, 51, 81, 293–94
L3, 52–53, 237
L5, 268
lumbar disc herniation/L4, 231–39
medications, 42–43
motor vehicle collision-associated,
    159, 160
in older adults, 62
people with limb loss, 234–35, 237
physical examination, 44
polyradiculopathy, 129, 138–39, 177–79
in pregnancy, 246, 251, 252
prevalence of, 40
prognosis, 45
recurrent, 173–82, 176t
spinal metastases-associated,
    122, 124–25
spinal stenosis and, 57–58, 62
surgery, 43–44, 73, 79, 175, 295
treatment, 53
upper lumbar, 53, 266–67, 266t
See also radiating leg pain
radiofrequency ablation (RFA), 26–27, 80